Fat To Gym Rat

Fat to Gym Rat

The Real Life Journey of Weight Loss

Lisa Virgil

NOTICE

The information in this book is not intended to substitute for any exercise or dietary program that may have been prescribed by your doctor. As with all exercise and dietary programs, you should get your doctor's approval before starting. Mention of specific products does not imply that they endorse this book. Internet addresses and phone numbers given in this book were accurate when it went to press.

Testimonials

"Fat to Gym Rat" is for those who are searching for the REAL life struggle of losing those unwanted pounds. Lisa has walked the walk and describes in depth the emotional, physical and mental struggles one will face while losing the pounds, to keep them off. This book is the perfect instruction book of HOW to lose the pounds, reality style. Lisa states it well in her book, "Do you want to lose weight now, or do you want to lose weight forever?" This is the last weight loss diet book you will ever read. Through Fat to Gym Rat you will discover who you are and who you want to become.

Dr. Candice Koch, BS, DC.

When I started Lisa's healthy lifestyle plan, I thought no way can I eat all this food and lose weight. I learned, from Lisa, that my eating habit of starving myself to lose weight was counter-productive because my body was storing fat. By following her plan, I lost 20 pounds and two pant sizes. The best part, though, is that I have kept it off for well over 18 months. I highly recommend "Fat to Gym Rat" to anyone who wants to lose weight by eating healthy, delicious food.

Dianne K. Price, Age 66

Lisa is a nutritionist and weight loss coach with a successful track record of accomplishing her goals through good-old-fashioned diet and exercise. No pills or gimmicks. Lisa's message is clear, and given our modern day society of miracle pills, fad diets, and ridiculous standards, her book needs to be out there reminding us of the core values of hard work and dedication.

Tanya Shaw

DEDICATION

This book is graciously dedicated to anyone who has the courage to begin their weight loss journey. May the path of success be laid clearly before your feet.

ACKNOWLEDGMENTS

Many thanks to all of the people on my "team" who have helped me along the way. I couldn't have done this without them.

Michael Valier, D.C. Family Chiropractic for challenging me to stick to my goal of health and encouraging me to never give up.

Jess Valier, D.C. Health Unlimited for helping me stay healthy and balanced through every step of my journey.

Parker Wells, CPT for his unfailing support, guidance, motivation, accountability and friendship.

Ivy Nadeau, LMT for undoing all of the hurt I put on my body and for her support and friendship.

AJ Virgil, Graphic Designer for my amazing book cover and his "hella good taste".

CONTENTS

Getting Started on Your Healthy Lifestyle

Common Concerns

Recipes

INTRODUCTION

THE JOURNEY OF A LIFETIME

...the wonderful, amazing, exhilarating, challenging, scary, inspiring, adventurous journey of losing weight and achieving your health and fitness goals. Weight loss is not an event; it is a personal journey. It is a journey that might have twists and turns, speed bumps, scenic routes, detours, and roadblocks, but a journey with views as breathtaking as Niagara Falls, as awe-inspiring as the Grand Canyon, and as incomparable as the Rocky Mountains. A journey that you will never forget.

I have taken this journey myself and am here to help guide and encourage you as you embark on your own personal journey. I know firsthand the highs and lows of the weight loss journey: the moments of frustration, despair, discouragement, fear, and heartbreak, as well as the sense of accomplishment, elation, pride, joy, and the victory of success. It wasn't always an easy journey, but it is a journey that I will never regret taking.

Yes, I was once teetering on the brink of morbid obesity, but now I embrace a healthy lifestyle. Like most people, I knew that I *needed* to change, but, like most people, I didn't know *how* to change. When I traveled on my weight loss journey I didn't have a map, compass, GPS, or tour-guide; I stumbled along on my own trying to find the best path. I learned a lot on the way, not only about nutrition, health, and fitness, but about myself.

Along the way, I met a lot of people like myself, people interested in becoming healthy, but not sure how to do it. They knew they needed to change the way they ate, but they were overwhelmed by the drastic dietary change most weight loss plans call for. They knew they needed to exercise, but they didn't know what exercises to do. As I went along, I realized that most of the people I met were not continuing on with me. I saw more and more people give up on their journey and I was greatly saddened by what I saw. I knew that if they had had a clearer path, success would have been in their grasp.

The clearer my path became, the more people would ask me how they could achieve success too. When people would ask me for advice, I could hear the hope in their voice. Hope for their own success. If I was standing before them telling them that I did it, they still had hope that they could do it too. They saw me reaching my goals and wanted to know what the "secret" was. There wasn't a "secret" where I could just say, "Do this," and they would achieve success. I realized, then, that I had the ability to help teach people how to make their own journeys successful. By taking what I had learned, I could encourage, instruct, and guide people on their own personal path to reach their health and fitness goals.

Losing weight is a process where you modify your thinking, eating, and activity levels, not just doing one "secret" thing. I have put together a road map of what real weight loss looks like: the highs and lows, the victories and failures, the setbacks and achievements. This is not a one-size-fits-all approach, it is not a quick-fix approach, and it is not an "instant results" approach; it is a realistic, gradual, achievable, lifelong approach that lets you be in control of your journey.

I will help teach you how to change the way you eat in a manner that will not overwhelm you. I will show you the emotional realities associated with losing weight. I will encourage you to embrace a healthy lifestyle. I will rejoice with you in your success. Welcome to the journey of a lifetime!

CHAPTER ONE

MY JOURNEY

HOW DID YOU DO IT?

"How did you do it?" is the inevitable question I get when people hear about my weight loss. When they hear my answer, their response is often a slightly disappointed "Oh." It took me awhile to figure out this somewhat puzzling reaction. Some people want me to answer that I had gastric bypass surgery and some want me to say I took a magic pill. If I had gastric bypass surgery, it justifies the people who think that they couldn't possibly lose weight without surgery. "Of course she lost weight, she had a gastric bypass. If I had a gastric bypass I could lose weight too." If I took a magic pill without having to do any work, they think it might work for them as well. "Magic pill! Sign me up!" The fact that I lost weight the "old-fashioned" way is a disappointment to many.

No one wants to hear that I changed my diet and started to eat healthy. Give up junk food? Unthinkable! The fact that I go to the gym and work out is a concept they don't want to consider. Cut into my TV time? Never! Everyone says they want to lose weight, yet no one wants to do what needs to be done to reach that goal. People don't want to have to work to achieve their goal of weight loss, they just want to *be* thinner.

When you see those infomercials for diet products that have amazing before and after photos, they usually don't tell you that it took a lot of hard work to get there. That they had to exercise and watch what they ate, even if the product they're promoting claims all you have to do is take their pill. Sometimes the ad for the "miracle" diet product will say in really small print that their product works "as part of a healthy diet and exercise program."

When you see a product that claims you can lose weight without having to change your diet or exercise, don't waste your money. If you are currently overweight and you don't change *anything* about how you eat or exercise, you will not lose weight. You *have* to change, so your weight will change.

As a society we have adapted an "instant" mentality. If we want to talk to someone we pull out our cell phone and expect the other person to answer immediately. If we're hungry we go to a fast food drive-thru and are eating before we pull away. If the computer takes more than 1.5 seconds to upload something we complain that it is slow. This mentality has crept into all aspects of our lives, including weight loss. So when people ask the other inevitable question—"How long did it take?"—they, once again, are disappointed by my response. "An entire year! That's way too long."

Never mind the fact that most people have struggled with their weight for years, perhaps their entire lives. You didn't wake up one morning suddenly twenty pounds overweight, so what makes you think you should be able to wake up one morning suddenly twenty pounds lighter? Is it because you see a commercial for a new diet pill that says, "Lose weight fast! Up to 13 pounds in one week!"? That type of weight loss is not healthy and it is usually not long term.

In the grand scheme of things, a year really isn't that long. Even though it took over a year to reach my final goal weight, it didn't take an entire year to see results. I lost 35 pounds and four pant sizes in the first four months and I had lost 50 pounds by eight months.

GROWING UP

As a young child I had always been fairly active. I started taking dance classes when I was four, just like all of the other little girls in the neighborhood. I would play outside for hours with my siblings and friends, riding bikes, jumping rope, playing hopscotch, and swinging on the swing set. In the summer we would walk to and from the local pool twice a day, once in the morning for swim lessons and again in the afternoon for hours of free swim. We spent most of our time outside making up games and going on imaginary adventures. The mantra we always heard was "go outside and play," and the ultimate cure for boredom was to "go clean your room."

I grew up in a small town in Wisconsin, the oldest of three children. My family lived in town until I was about seven years old and then we moved to the country. In Wisconsin, if you live in the country that does not mean the suburbs; it means either you live on a dairy farm or next to a dairy farm.

My brother had a blast playing at the neighbor's dairy farm all day with the neighbor's two boys, but there was no one for my sister and me to play with except each other. For a while, we would play together, but once we reached a certain age you didn't "play" anymore; you "hung out" and listened to music and did "big kid" stuff. I loved to read, so most of my day was spent lying in bed reading through a stack of books while my sister listened to music.

Even though we became less active during the day, my sister and I would still go to dance class once a week. I really enjoyed the dance classes, and we would travel to Minnesota every year to compete in a big dance competition. Dance classes went from once a week to a couple of times a week. Which lead us to eventually move back into town, conveniently around the corner from the dance studio.

I would spend hours dancing, annoying my teachers by practicing my steps while sitting at my desk at school, irritating my mom by dancing in the aisles of the grocery store, making my dance teacher proud because I always knew my routines. I started to clean the dance studio to pay for my dance lessons, so I would get extra time to practice in front of the mirrors before I had to start cleaning.

As I got older, I started to help teach some of the classes. I would go straight from school to the dance studio, where I would stay until it was late in the evening. I would spend more of my waking hours at the dance studio than I would at home. The innumerable hours of dancing, more often than not in tap shoes with a heel, started to take its toll on me. I started to suffer excruciating knee pain in both knees. What had always been a joy to me suddenly became a burden. I would strap on my tap shoes with dread, knowing I would be spending my evening suffering through intense pain. The pain eventually got to the point where I needed to see my doctor, who quickly sent me to see an orthopedic surgeon. After some x-rays and an exam, it was determined that I would need knee surgery on not just one, but on both of my knees.

As I recovered from the first surgery, I didn't know what to do with myself. I had always thought of myself as a dancer. Everyone around me knew me as a dancer. Instead of seeing the knee surgery as a bump in the road, I saw it as a dead end to my dancing. By the time I had surgery on the second knee, I had resigned myself to the fact that dancing was something I wouldn't do again.

A few short weeks after my second knee surgery, just barely off the crutches, I moved to Colorado to be a nanny. I went from being an active dancer to someone recovering from an injury sitting around taking care of a newborn. So began the decline in my activity levels and the increase in my weight.

Within two years of moving to Colorado I was happily married and eagerly anticipating the birth of my first child. The upcoming arrival of the first grandchild on both mine and my husband's side was a momentous occasion. I thrived in the role of expectant mother and eagerly watched my belly grow.

When my baby was born, it definitely changed my activity levels. Sedentary was an understatement. I did the things that moms do. I spent hours and hours just holding the baby, enjoying every moment. Delighting in every baby accomplishment, the adorable little baby sounds, the smiles, the dimples in elbows and knees, the soft baby skin, and the wonderful baby smell. I played peek-a-boo and pat-a-cake, changed diapers, watched Sesame Street, gave hugs and kisses, washed laundry, took tons of pictures, gave baths, and called grandma to brag about how wonderful the baby was. Nowhere on the list of "things moms do" was exercise and take care of herself.

While I hadn't gained too much weight when I was pregnant, I most certainly did not weigh what I weighed before I was pregnant. Add on four more babies and you can see where weighing more after each baby could become a problem. The combination of multiple pregnancies, poor diet, and a sedentary lifestyle kept my weight climbing. By the time I had my fifth child my weight was alarming, but I was so far entrenched in "mommy-mode" I didn't even think about my weight.

I was a busy stay-at-home, homeschooling mom. My whole life was my home and my children. My children were happy and my home was happy. My children loved me even though I was overweight, because that is the only way they ever knew me, and my husband didn't love me less because I was overweight. So what difference did it make?

Unlike a lot of people who are overweight, I never did yo-yo diets. I tried one diet, just once. The ten pounds I lost on that diet quickly came back and brought along fifteen more pounds to keep them company around my bulging waistline. So I guess I did a "yo" diet. When I tried that diet and failed, it scared me. I had heard stories of people who kept losing and regaining weight, getting heavier and heavier each time. I didn't want to get any heavier, so I figured if I didn't try another diet I wouldn't get any heavier. Turns out that wasn't such a good plan.

I never really tried to diet as I got heavier, but I did try to get fit a couple of times. An exercise video not too long after the birth of my first child that was quickly pushed aside and forgotten due to the demands of parenthood. A membership at a women's only gym that I had to give up when we moved to a small town that didn't have a gym I could transfer my membership to. One workout with a friend that was supposed to be the first of many, but ended abruptly when we both found out we were pregnant a couple weeks later. A membership at a gym that my husband said was too expensive so I had to cancel it the next day. A treadmill for Christmas that my daughter got her hair wound up in within a few hours of setting up, so it was deemed dangerous and sat gathering dust.

My half hearted attempts at fitness didn't get me very far and my fear of diets didn't help the situation very much. It seemed to me that it was easier to just let things be as they were, enjoying my family and food and forgetting about fitness. And so I did.

BEGINNING OF THE BATTLE

In February 2007 I went shopping and to dinner with a friend. My friend and I had a great time, despite the nagging sore throat that had started halfway through the evening. Thinking that I might be coming down with a cold, I took some pain relievers when I got home and went to bed.

In the night, I rolled over and was seized by a wave of vertigo that left me in a cold sweat. The nausea was a punch to the belly. As the intensity of the spinning finally slowed down, the realization of my dilemma set in. I had just rolled onto my side facing the inside of the bed, but the nausea was telling me I was going to need the bathroom, soon. I needed to roll back over and get out of bed and make it to the bathroom while the room was wildly spinning. I cautiously rolled over, but the vertigo didn't care how cautious I was. My trip to the bathroom no longer fell into the "soon" category; it fell into the "now" category.

I was afraid to move and afraid of what would happen if I didn't move. It was time for some serious back-up. Luckily for me, there was some readily available in the form of my husband, if only I could open my mouth to speak without my last meal joining me in the bed. "Honey..." I managed to croak. No response. I tried again.

"Honey... help." It's amazing how the word "help" roused my husband from an earth-shatteringly loud-snoring deep sleep to wakefulness in a millisecond. He jolted straight up in bed saying, "What?" All I could manage was one word. "Dizzy." My husband was instantly by my side. "What do you need?" In a more coherent state I could have suggested something like, "Wash the bedding after I throw up," but I answered with "Bathroom." Now, at any other time, my one-word responses would be greatly appreciated by my husband, but, for now, concern over-shadowed appreciation.

So began an almost three-year battle that would change my life in ways I never could have predicted. I was no stranger to dizziness. I had suffered bouts of dizziness off and on for over ten years. I'm prone to a condition called Benign Positional Paroxysmal Vertigo (BPPV). BPPV is an occurrence of deposits getting displaced into the equilibrium regulating part of the ear. As the deposits bounce around the inner ear, they send conflicting signals to your brain as to where your body is in relation to space. The conflicting information the brain receives results in the sensation of your body spinning, commonly referred to as vertigo.

In the past, several different things have triggered episodes of BPPV. Once, one of my children bonked their head into mine and that triggered an episode. Sometimes a change in altitude would not make me just need to "pop" my ears; it would trigger my BPPV. Other times illness would trigger it, just like it did in this case. My seemingly innocent sore throat was not so innocent. The inflammation in my throat caused pressure to build up in my ear, triggering my dizzy nightmare. Anything that causes me to have pressure in my ear could potentially cause an episode of BPPV.

BPPV is a fairly common, easily-remedied condition. The head is manipulated in a series of movements, called the Epley Maneuver, to re-position the deposits back into the part of the ear where they belong. After having numerous episodes of BPPV in the past, I wasn't overly alarmed when it happened. I assumed I would go to the physical therapist, have them perform the Epley Maneuver, do some vestibular and balance therapy, and I would feel better. Wrong. I went to the physical therapist, who performed the Epley Maneuver and did the vestibular and balance therapy, but I didn't get better. Hey, didn't my BPPV get the memo? I was supposed to get better.

The constant dizziness and accompanying nausea kept me immobilized. I was unable to drive or do many of my normal day-to-day tasks. I had intense photophobia. No, that is not a fear of getting my picture taken; it is an extreme sensitivity to light. I was unable to tolerate any light at all: fluorescent lights, incandescent lights, flashlights, sunlight all had me cringing in pain. I had a constant shimmering and flickering in my vision and episodes of double vision. Every time I closed my eyes I would see flashes of light similar to a strobe light. The strobe light effect caused me to get disco music stuck in my head. Great. Now I'm dizzy and I feel like watching 'Saturday Night Fever.'

I felt like my eyes were trying to hold the world together, but they just couldn't do it. The constant strain on my eyes caused a tremendous amount of eye fatigue that would trigger unrelenting headaches. After a handful of doctors and numerous tests to rule out all the scary stuff, I got a little relief from one of my medications. Such a ray of hope to not be paralyzed by dizziness and nausea! But that was all that happened. How anti-climatic.

All of my other symptoms were still as severe, and the dizziness and nausea were still there, just not at a paralyzing level. Instead of the intense spinning sensation, my dizziness felt more like a constant feeling of lightheadedness or a swimming sensation, like I was under water. The nausea became a continuously queasy feeling combined with that weird feeling you get in the pit of your stomach when you're in an elevator that stops suddenly. Still more doctors, prescribing increasingly powerful medications with serious side effects. My husband desperately searching the Internet for possible causes to my mysterious debilitating illness, but never finding an answer. I didn't have MS, I didn't have a brain tumor, I didn't have fibromyalgia, and I was fairly confident I wasn't crazy.

The strain on me was tremendous. Every day was a battle for survival. I was trying hard to maintain some semblance of normalcy for our family, but it was extremely difficult. The simplest tasks were no longer simple. Anything involving motion, either me moving or me seeing movement, would cause my symptoms to worsen. Suddenly the once joyous task of cooking became a dreaded chore. Stirring or mixing something would cause intense vertigo and nausea. The sight of boiling water made me physically ill. If we were watching a movie as a family I spent most of the movie with my eyes closed because I couldn't tolerate watching the movement on the screen. Even watching my children play was difficult. The sight of a crayon moving back and forth as they colored, watching them chase each other around, and the constant call of "Mom, watch this!" now were things that caused me to feel overwhelmed with dizziness instead of maternal pride.

Our family adapted to my illness as best it could. Unable to tolerate light, I would cook by candlelight and we would eat in semi-darkness. My husband would say, "A romantic dinner for seven," and wink at me across the table. At least I *think* he was winking at me. The house was kept as dark as possible and the kids started to think I might be a vampire. I would wear sunglasses inside, which totally mortified the kids when we were in public, but it was something I had to do. If I didn't wear the sunglasses I wouldn't be able to open my eyes. The fluorescent lights were the worst because they were not only light, but flickering light, and that was something my eyes just couldn't tolerate. I told the kids I was practicing to be a movie star, but they never believed me.

In September 2009 the tremendous stress on my body and the never-ending strain on my eyes caused me to lose my sight. It was a terrifying, sobering symptom. When I lost my sight it wasn't like

I couldn't see anything at all and everything was black like when your eyes are closed. Instead, what I saw was a blur of colors where nothing could be defined. I would hear one of my children talk to me and see an undefined mass of color instead of my child. I couldn't see their eyes, nose, or mouth, just a lighter color than the color that was their body, which was a blob of color without limbs. The thought of never seeing my children again left a hole in my heart. To not see my only daughter walk down the aisle when she got married, to not see another touchdown, soccer goal or wrestling match from my boys, to not see the beautiful work of art one of the kids had created, just for me, was too much to bear.

When I lost my sight I felt I had three options: One, I was going to be blind. Two, I was going to die from an undiagnosed brain tumor. Three, I was going to get healthy. An emergency visit with my eye doctor, who found nothing physically wrong with my eyes except extreme eye fatigue, followed by yet another brain MRI which, once again, showed no sign of a tumor, left me with my final option. So the only thing left was for me to get healthy.

I decided that I had suffered long enough and I would take my health into my own hands. I created an action plan which I thought would help me reach my goals and got to work.

FIGHTING BACK

My mom had been encouraging (nagging) me to try chiropractic care for a while and I finally decided to give it a chance. I figured that what I had been trying wasn't working, so I needed to try something else. I added chiropractic care to my action plan, did some research, and found a chiropractor that looked like he could help me. I was looking to get healthy and here was a doctor that actually looked like he practiced what he preached. I was a little nervous about getting my back "cracked," but I felt I needed to give it a try. Besides, then my mom would quit hassling me.

My chiropractor was very thorough and professional and seemed to be genuinely concerned about my health. I told him I wanted to get healthy and had created an action plan to reach that goal. He asked if he could have a copy to look at. After he reviewed it, he did the unthinkable. He asked me about my weight. Oh my. This was the fourteenth doctor/medical professional I had gone to since the onset of my illness, but he was the first to even mention my weight. He did it in a very non-judgmental, matter-of-fact way. It wasn't like, "You're pretty huge, maybe you should cut back on the cookies." It was more like, "I saw you had something about diet on your action plan." Yes, I did have something on my action plan about diet. Little did I know how it would change my life.

I started going to the chiropractor three times a week. Thankfully, the adjustments were not as scary as I had thought they would be. The chiropractor always told me exactly what he was going to do so I would know what to expect. If a wave of dizziness came over me, he would wait until it passed before continuing with my adjustment. Once my adjustments started to hold, my daily headaches and episodes of dizziness improved.

Then I got LASIK surgery on my eyes. Apparently there was a drastic difference between the sight of my right eye and left eye and that can cause double vision. The LASIK surgery corrected my double vision and eased almost all of my eye fatigue. What an amazing thing to not only be able to see again, but to see without the glasses or contacts I had been wearing for over twenty-five years. My sight is such a precious gift, and I was so thankful to have it back.

Eventually, I was diagnosed with two types of migraine variants. The first migraine variant is Persistent Aura Without Infarction, which would cause me to have a migraine aura where I would see the shimmering and flashing lights and caused my extreme sensitivity to light. And, as its name suggests, it was definitely persistent. I was also diagnosed with Vertiginous Migraine, which is a dizzy migraine, and that (surprise, surprise!) would cause my dizziness and nausea.

I am also the victim of a Dysfunctional Vestibular System. The vestibular system is the brain, eyes, and inner ear working together to receive and process sensory information regarding our position in space. Since my ears kept sending crazy dizzy messages to my brain, my brain decided to stop listening to my ears and tried to get all of its sensory input from my eyes. So when I felt like my eyes were trying to hold the world together, they really were. My inability to correctly process sensory information continually causes me to struggle with dizziness, so I guess I really *am* a dizzy blonde.

As things finally started to fall into place, I felt ready to move on to the next level of health. Instead of just having improvement in my symptoms, I wanted to really *be* healthy. I had put together my action plan, but I wasn't really sure how someone *became* healthy.

REALITY CHECK

Over the years of my illness I had never really looked in a mirror or objectively appraised the way I looked. I was too busy just trying to survive my day-to-day demands. My lack of physical fitness and my actual weight were horrifying. I had deluded myself into thinking I was still fit because I ran around after my five children. What do you mean that doesn't count?

I hadn't looked in a full-length mirror in years, so it was easy to pretend I wasn't as big as I really was. Me, heavy? Nah. There are a lot of companies out there geared towards making women feel better by making their sizes much larger than "normal" sizes. A size 10 in one brand might be a size 14 in another brand. If you know what brand to buy you can delude yourself quite well. "Look at me, size 12, just like Marilyn Monroe."

I had always felt that since I didn't need to buy my clothes at a plus-size store, I was still okay. Then my mom took me shopping for some new clothes for my birthday. We went to several stores, but eventually ended up at a plus-size store. The new clothes weren't as exciting when I had to go to a special store to buy them because regular clothes wouldn't fit me anymore.

I had stopped weighing myself when I reached 180 pounds. At 4'11", 180 pounds, size 2X in shirts, and size 16 in pants, I had to face the cold hard reality of my obesity. It was so embarrassing to admit to myself how fat I had actually become. I felt like a terrible person with no self-control, no self-discipline, no self-respect, and no self-esteem.

It would have been easy for me to give in to depression and let it wrap itself around me and protect me from my reality, but I had come too far. The thought of my illness and the tremendous toll it took on me outweighed my feelings of self-loathing and embarrassment. I had to keep working towards my goal of health.

Getting Started

When I started, like most overweight people, the thought of going to a gym filled me with terror. The thought of working out where other people could see me was kind of like that nightmare where you're in public and you forgot to put on your pants. I knew it was not something I could do. Instead, I pulled out the exercise bike I already owned, got some new music on my iPod, and got to work.

At first, all I could do was ten minutes on the bike. Really? It was difficult to think of ten minutes of physical activity as the most I could do, but, nonetheless, it was all I could manage. I'd huff, puff, sweat like crazy, and pray I wouldn't have a heart attack for those agonizing ten minutes. I slowly built up to 45 minutes, but my poor bottom was starting to seriously protest all that time on the bike. Ouch.

I splurged and got a 10-minute incremental hip-hop aerobics DVD. Dancing was something that I had always loved, but I hadn't thought about it in twenty years. Remembering how much I had enjoyed dancing as a young girl, I thought the hip-hop DVD would be fun. Ten minutes with the smiling girl on the DVD and I was hooked. My bedroom became my workout room and my exercise DVD collection grew. Heaven help the poor soul who tried to interrupt my workout!

While I felt like I was getting in shape, I wasn't sure if I was losing any weight. I hadn't weighed myself since the mind-blowing 180 pounds. One day though, I noticed my watch was too loose, then my bra was loose, and then my belt was loose...maybe I had lost weight? I had lost 5 pounds! That small taste of victory was all I needed. The first 20 pounds came off easily when I finally started to lose. The next 15 came off steadily at 1-1.5 pounds a week. Losing 35 pounds in four months was an amazing thing. The store became my playground. "What size do I need this week?" I would think as I happily skipped to the smaller and smaller sizes.

Then the dreaded plateau stalled me out. I knew I had to do something different if I wanted to reach the weight loss goals I had set for myself, but what? My son encouraged me to try lifting weights so I could tone up, not just lose fat. My response: "Lift weights!?! I'm a girl! I don't know how to lift weights. That's crazy talk!" When I got done freaking out about the possibility of lifting weights, I evaluated where I was at in my weight loss journey. As much as I hated to admit it, I had gone as far as I could at home on my own. I decided I had to put aside my insecurities and try a gym. I needed help, and the best place to find it was at a gym with a personal trainer.

Oh, lucky day for the membership counselor at the gym! Talk about an easy sell. I had my gym bag packed and I was ready to go. All-access pass? Sure! Three session personal training package? You bet! Add another ten session personal training package on for a discount? Now we're talking! Reward program?

Why not! The membership counselor gave me the grand tour of the gym and I put my gym bag in a locker and got on a treadmill.

Now, while the membership counselor had had an easy sell on my membership, I was still struggling with my insecurities and the thought of people looking at me. Luckily, I had chosen to come to the gym on a Saturday night so it wasn't very crowded. As I was walking on the treadmill I noticed a police officer walking through the gym. Then I noticed a couple more police officers by the front desk. "Wow, our city police officers take their health seriously," I thought to myself. Then I noticed the paramedics. What the heck was going on? I casually looked around the gym, and not one person was paying attention to the police or the paramedics. The people on treadmills, bikes, and elliptical machines kept up their pace, the people lifting weights kept doing their sets, and no one paid attention to the drama unfolding amongst them.

My shoulders sagged with relief. If no one even paid attention to the police and paramedics, then they wouldn't pay attention to me either. My journey toward health and fitness began in earnest. I went to the gym to walk on the treadmill, but was still extremely intimidated by all of the equipment. Everything looked complicated, and all of the people using the equipment seemed to know what they were doing.

Then came my first personal training session. I had spoken to my trainer on the phone to schedule our first meeting, and I was both nervous and excited to get started. On our first session my trainer took a complete medical history, and we talked about what goals I wanted to reach. Then he took me around the gym and got me started on those "not-as-intimidating-with-my-trainer" pieces of equipment. He wrote everything down for me so I could do it again on my own, explaining what all of the numbers and exercises were as we went. There was no looking back; I was on my way to becoming a full-fledged gym rat.

JUST DIVE IN

While my trainer and I set goals and worked hard, my weight stayed on that agonizing plateau. After eight excruciatingly long weeks with my weight not changing, I knew I had to do that one thing I had been dreading. My chiropractor had told me I should do it months earlier and my trainer agreed with him.

I had tried to do it, I really did, but I couldn't bring myself to do it. I had gotten ready to do it, but I had just sat paralyzed in the locker room. Now I realized that no matter how much I didn't *want* to do it, I *needed* to do it. I felt physically ill just thinking about it, but I could no longer put it off. I put on my swimsuit and forced myself out of the safety of the locker room. I felt like I was going to die for a few seconds, but when I started to breathe again I realized I would be okay. I was in my swimsuit, in a public setting where other people could see me, but I wasn't going to die; I could do it.

I got in the water and then was like "Now what?" Did I even remember how to swim? Was it like riding a bike, where I would remember once I got started? Or would I start, and then slowly sink to the bottom of the pool when I realized I had forgotten how to keep myself afloat? There was only one way to find out, and I was already in the pool. I pushed off the wall and, to my delight, I didn't sink to the bottom, but successfully made my way across the entire length of the pool. Just like the hip-hop DVD, I was instantly hooked.

Weightlessness! What an amazing feeling! The pool became my new friend, one I would spend countless hours with. Now, before you jump to the conclusion that I'm some kind of accomplished swimmer, let me assure you that is the furthest thing from the truth. I can't do the front crawl, I don't flip around under water at the edge of the pool, I don't time myself, I don't wear goggles or a swim cap, I don't even put my head under the water, and once someone at the gym told me I swam very "relaxed," which I'm pretty sure meant "slow."

I do, however, do a modified breaststroke with a technique that would make any real swimmer cringe, use the kick board if I really want to work my glutes, do the doggie paddle when I want to burn a billion calories, and I most definitely swim 4-5 times a week. The solitude, peace, and relaxation I achieve while I'm swimming followed by the unbeatable endorphin rush is a winning combination in my book. It's like the salty and sweet of workouts, totally addictive.

SHAKE YOUR GROOVE THING

After doing the hip-hop DVD I realized how much I still really enjoyed dancing. The twenty years since I had last danced had gone by quickly, but even quicker was the return of my love of dance. I didn't own a leotard, jazz shoes, tights, leg warmers, or tap shoes anymore, and the routines that I had once been able to dance in my sleep were long faded from memory, but the happiness and joy I felt when I danced was the same as it had been all those years ago. While I enjoyed lifting weights and swimming at the gym, my favorite cardio was dancing.

At the gym there was an exercise room where they offered a variety of classes, including Zumba, which my trainer encouraged me to try. I had heard Zumba was fun and it was like dancing, so I thought I'd give it a try. I got to the class and found a spot in the safety of the back of the room, only to realize that the entire wall was made of glass and the class was exposed to the rest of the gym. My stomach tightened up and I felt extremely nervous at the thought of dancing where other people could see me. Dancing at home behind the safety of a closed door was a lot different.

I tried to relax and listen to the instructor, but I noticed a guy in the gym just standing and watching the class. I completely shut down. I felt like I was going to cry or have a nervous breakdown. I wanted to leave, but felt like more people would look at me if I left in the middle of the class. I tried to follow along, but I was paralyzed. The nice lady in front of me tried to encourage me by telling me to "just keep moving." Little did she know how impossible that was for me.

Finally, the class came to an end and I was able to leave the gym. I was shaking and sweating and weak. I was so glad it was over. It felt like everyone in the gym was looking at me. My struggles with self-esteem were brought to the surface, and it made me feel vulnerable, a feeling I really don't like. I decided to stick with dancing in the safety of my room where I knew no one could see.

Then, one day, I noticed this young guy who would break dance in the exercise room when there weren't any classes. It totally fascinated me. He didn't care if people looked at him; he was just doing his own thing. Nobody seemed to be watching him, except me. I would watch him discreetly while I worked out. I wondered if he was a dance teacher; maybe I could take some private lessons.

I wanted to dance, but I was afraid. The thought of being looked at made me extremely uncomfortable, but my love of dance continued to pull on me. The room full of mirrors beckoned me, and I could no longer resist. It felt safer to have someone with me, so my daughter came with me for moral support. She knew I wanted to dance, but was too afraid to do it on my own. We went to dance when the exercise room was empty, so it would just be the two of us. She was totally relaxed, dancing with abandon and the exuberance of youth. I was stiff and tense and consumed with self-consciousness.

I glanced out of the room and saw someone watching us. Just like the Zumba class, I totally shut down. My daughter encouraged me to ignore the onlooker and dance some more. "Who cares if they're watching, Mom?" she said to me. "I care," was my answer. "Well, you shouldn't care," she replied swiftly. In an effort to get me to relax she started dancing like a goofball, doing the most ridiculous moves and making funny faces. It definitely made me laugh, but it wasn't enough to get me to dance. I was trying to gather our things so we could leave when the young break-dancer came in to dance.

I told him we were just leaving so he could have the room to himself, but he encouraged us to stay and dance with him. We ended up talking for a while and he agreed to teach us a few moves the next time we came to the gym. I was so excited about learning some hip-hop dance moves that I completely forgot about being embarrassed or self-conscious.

Soon my dancing friend and I became a fixture at the gym. Dancing between me and any potential onlookers, he became my security blanket. I figured if anyone was watching they would obviously be watching him and his impressive dance moves, not even bothering to look at me. So I slowly began to gain more confidence. Sometimes other dancers would join us. They would work on their routines and I would mess around doing my own dancing, using them as a wall of protection.

Sometimes I would feel like dancing, but if there were no other dancers to use as my security blanket or wall of protection I would do the elliptical instead. Sigh. As my New Year's resolution I decided I would find the courage to "dance like no one's watching." Little did I know how quickly that would happen.

One night I went to the gym, looking eagerly at the exercise room to see if any dancers were there. Darn. Not one dancer. Resigning myself to the fact that it would be me and the elliptical, I stalled by talking to one of my numerous friends at the gym. I mentioned how disappointed I was that no other dancers were there that evening, because I had really wanted to dance. My friend challenged me to dance by myself. She knew my New Year's resolution and called me on it.

I tried to defer, but she was insistent. She walked me to the exercise room and refused to leave until I started to dance. My heart was pounding and my stomach was in knots, but one look at her face confirmed that she was resolute. She stood with her arms crossed in front of her chest, daring me to do what I had challenged myself to do. With my fingers sweating and shaking I turned on my iPod and put the earbuds in. When the music started, so did I. Satisfied that I had begun, my friend left me to dance.

There was no turning back. With the music blaring in my ears, effectively tuning out all outside noise, I was in my own little world. Just me and my music. I'm not sure if I "danced like no one was watching," but I danced by myself. It was a huge turning point for me. All of my years of low self-esteem and extreme self-consciousness slowly started to fade. So what if I wasn't the best dancer? I enjoyed it and it made me happy, so I stopped worrying about everyone else and what they might be thinking, and focused on what was important to me.

CHAPTER TWO

THE EMOTIONAL SIDE OF WEIGHT LOSS

ALL ABOUT YOU

Weight loss is an extremely personal decision, and I mean that in a very literal way. Weight loss is a decision you make in your head that, in turn, creates a behavioral change. Weight loss happens first in your head, then in your body. Most people don't realize this. I know I didn't. "What do you mean weight loss happens in your head?" people ask me. I mean that your thinking, your mentality, your whole perspective needs to change.

Whenever you hear about someone who has experienced significant weight loss, they can invariably tell you *exactly* when they reached their turning point. They don't say they just happened to lose weight, or they're not sure how they lost weight. They will tell you that they had an epiphany, or that something scared, upset, motivated, or inspired them enough to make them change their thinking. That is how weight loss happens in your head.

I talk to a lot of people about weight loss and health, and can often tell by talking to them whether or not they have reached the point where their attempts will result in long-term success, or if they haven't mentally made the commitment to lifelong change. If they have truly reached the point where they are willing to surrender their former way of life and embrace a healthy new lifestyle. If they have decided that they want to lose weight more than anything.

People might think they want to lose weight more than anything until they start to realize exactly what that means. They want to lose weight, but they don't want to give up the convenience of fast food restaurants. They want to lose weight, but they want to go to the movies once a week and eat five pounds of buttered popcorn and two pounds of candy with their diet soda. They want to lose weight, but they want to go out for lunch with everyone at the office three times a week. They want to lose weight, but they want to guzzle down a few beers with their wings and nachos while they cheer for their favorite team. They want to lose weight, but they don't want to actually have to cook something. They want to lose weight, but they don't want to change how they eat. They want to lose weight, but they don't want to change their lifestyle. They want to lose weight, but they want everything to stay the same.

If you're reading this book, you're definitely thinking about making a change in your life. Maybe you want to lose a few pounds for a wedding or class reunion. Maybe you've been told you're pre-diabetic and you need to change your diet. Maybe you've recently lost a parent and that scares you. Maybe you're morbidly obese and you think gastric bypass surgery is your only solution. Maybe you're tired of always being the "fat one" in a social gathering. Maybe you feel exhausted trying to keep up with your daily demands because of your weight. Maybe you're afraid you're going to die. Whatever the reason, educating yourself is always a positive thing.

HAVE YOU DECIDED?

Have you decided to lose weight? Have you reached the point where you are willing to do *whatever* it takes to get healthy? Can you tell me *exactly* what brought you to the point where you said, "Enough is enough"? Have you even *reached* the point where you have said, "Enough is enough"? Do you *believe* you can lose weight and be healthy? Are you *really* ready to change? Are you going to do this or not? Decide!

You might have a stack of twelve books on fitness, health, nutrition, or diet that tell you twelve different things and you don't know what to think. Now, I'm not a doctor, trainer or registered dietician. I'm just a regular person who happened to turn her life around. All I can do is tell you how I did it and what worked for me. How I did it was not rocket science, it wasn't cutting-edge information or technology, it wasn't a miracle. It was a *decision*. I decided that I was going to get healthy, and I did. Now that might sound simple and you might be thinking, "I decided I wanted to lose weight and be healthy, but nothing happened." But did you really?

When you decide you want Chinese for dinner, you go out and get it. When you decide what movie you want to see, you go watch it. When you decide what you want to wear, you go put it on. When you decide what book you want, you go read it. What do you do when you decide to lose weight? Ummmm...

Do you read a diet book? Do you go to the doctor for advice? Do you look up the latest diet trend on the internet? Do you try the latest "miracle drug"? Do you try a weight loss program offered through a local gym? Do you eat only cabbage soup? Do you do what your friend's sister's acupuncturist's cousin did? Do you get help from a nutritionist? Do you order the latest exercise equipment you see on an infomercial? Do you get a personal trainer? Do you tell yourself you're going to eat healthy all week? Do you purge your cabinets? Do you swear off junk food for the rest of your life? Do you try surgery? Do you say you'll start on Monday?

Most people will get a diet book and check out what's on the internet. They might go down the "weight loss" aisle at the drugstore to see if there's an "instant" pill. Perhaps they'll spend some money on a home gym and swear that they won't eat junk food this week. Listen eagerly to what their friend's sister's acupuncturist's cousin did. Do a little research on gastric bypass surgery. Promise themselves that they will start on Monday...

WHY WAIT?

Why wait until Monday to start getting healthy? There is no rule that says you can't start right now. I'm not sure why everyone thinks Monday is the best day to start a new exercise or eating plan. Mondays tend to be hectic and stressful, so why would you choose your busiest day to try something new? Start on Friday and you'll have your whole weekend to make healthy choices, and you'll be three days ahead of all the people who waited until Monday. Start on your least busy day, start on your lunch break, start right after work, start right now! What are you waiting for, Monday?

Most people will not get advice from their doctor, because that takes too long. They won't get help from a nutritionist because they can read a diet book or look up diet information on the internet. They won't try a program at a local gym because they want to try their "miracle pill" first. And who needs a personal trainer when you have a home gym?

What is your decision going to look like? Are you visual, so you set up an action plan? Methodical, so you research all the weight loss programs before choosing one that's right for you? Are you spontaneous, so you sign up at the gym closest to your house? Logical, so you make a pros and cons list of all of your options before making a decision? Passionate, so you jump in with both feet? Timid, so you want someone to do it with you? Are you ready for the biggest adventure of your life? Then *decide*, and do it!

I had decided that enough was enough; my health came first. Before everything. Period. If I didn't take care of myself no one else was going to. Taking care of myself meant less time taking care of my family, and that was something my family wasn't used to. I had been a stay-at-home, homeschooling mom since my kids were born. My kids were used to instant access to me 24 hours a day, seven days a week, 365 days a year, and suddenly that was different.

IT'S ALL ABOUT YOU

Once, when I was working with my trainer, another trainer congratulated my trainer on how good I was doing with my weight loss. My trainer was quick to respond that he hadn't done it, I had. There are 168 hours in a week; I work with my trainer for only one of those hours. I lost the weight, my trainer didn't. He was there to help encourage, motivate, instruct, and guide me, but he couldn't lose weight for me. Weight loss is all about you. It's your decision and your responsibility. I can't lose weight for you. A trainer can't lose weight for you. An online program can't lose weight for you. A miracle pill can't lose weight for you. *You* have to lose weight for you.

If I had continued on the path I was on, I have no doubt I would have been dead within five years, and then what would have happened? Who would take care of my kids if I was gone? I had to continue on my journey and hope my kids would eventually understand that I had to get healthy so I would be there for them.

Some people will try to get healthy for someone else, but I had to do it for myself. If I had tried to do it for someone else I would resent them when I was hungry, felt deprived, or was so sore I could hardly walk after a difficult workout. Yes, I wanted to be there for my children but it wasn't just for them. I was doing it because *I* wanted to watch them grow up. *I* wanted to see them experience all that life has to offer. *I* wanted to celebrate all of life's joys with them. My kids would grow up, get married, have their own families, and experience life even if I died due to a weight-related health issue, but *I* wanted to be there to see it all.

It was hard trying to find the right balance between taking care of myself and reaching the goals I had set, and meeting the demands of my family. Some things I just couldn't do anymore. I couldn't sit around and watch television with my kids anymore. I couldn't watch television in general; being bombarded with commercials for food every few minutes when you're trying to lose weight just doesn't work. Go figure.

Trying to fit my workouts into an already jam-packed schedule of five children, husband, homeschooling, cooking, cleaning, laundry, and kids' activities wasn't very easy. I got very adept at ignoring the dishes in the sink and the laundry that needed to be folded. Trust me; every time I came home from the gym the dishes and the laundry were waiting patiently for me.

UNDERLYING OBSTACLES

You need to understand yourself: what motivates you, what encourages you, what scares you. You need to deal with emotional/comfort eating, compulsive/stress eating, self-image/self-esteem, dependent/addictive behavior patterns, self-abuse, and any other underlying issues that could be contributing to your weight. Some people have gastric bypass surgery and lose weight only to gain it right back because they haven't changed their thinking or resolved their emotional issues.

I had always thought I didn't have any emotional issues contributing to my weight. I would say the reason I was heavy was because I really enjoyed my cooking, which was true, but there were underlying emotional issues I was never aware of. Yep, I was the Queen of Denial. Just give me a crown and scepter and let me float down that river.

I had serious issues with comfort and stress eating. Whatever I needed, there was a type of food to fit my needs. Food that reminded me of my childhood, food that helped me forget, food that gave me something to do when I was anxious, food to help me celebrate, food to show others that I cared about them, food to show that I was a great cook, food to help me pass the time, food for watching television, food that looked good on television, food just because I felt like eating, food when I was scared, and food when I was happy. Food was a great friend, always by my side.

When I was finally honest with myself about my relationship with food, I was able to change my relationship with it. Now, my relationship with food didn't change overnight. It wasn't like, "Food, I know we've had a lot of fun in the past, but I think I should start eating differently. No, it's not you, it's me. I will always love you." It was an awareness of the emotions tied to the food I was eating, and how I felt about what I was eating, and trying to separate the food from the emotions.

I know there are a lot of people who think they don't have any emotional issues contributing to their weight, just like I did. It's embarrassing to think of yourself as emotionally weak or somehow emotionally dysfunctional. Some people will be quick to point the finger of blame at their slow thyroid, their fat family tree, their PCOS, the three kids they've given birth to, the high cost of healthy food in relation to their budget, their back pain that renders them incapable of working out, or any other excuse that they can think of to convince themselves and the people around them that their weight doesn't have an emotional component. Trying to blame your weight on anything you can think of that sounds even remotely valid will not help you lose weight.

Losing weight is a highly emotional process. It's not as simple as "If I eat less calories then I use I will lose weight." It is facing your relationship with food. For some people their relationship with food is very complex with many layers of emotional issues. For some, it may even involve dealing with an abusive relationship from their past. If your emotional issues are significant, complex, or just downright overwhelming it may be a good idea to get some outside help sorting through them.

Dealing with your emotional issues with regard to your weight is not a sign of weakness. Admitting you need help is a tremendous show of strength and courage. Pretending you don't have a problem is far less courageous than facing the problem head on. So don't pretend you don't have any emotional issues dealing with food. Be honest with yourself no matter how painful or embarrassing it is.

For some people, admitting they have an emotional issue tied to their weight and dealing with that issue will be the hardest part of their weight loss journey. As I will tell you repeatedly throughout this book, take your time dealing with each step. Don't feel like you have to race to the finish line; take your time and do what you need to do to achieve success. If you need to get counseling to deal with an abusive past relationship in order to get your relationship with food going in the right direction, that is obviously going to take longer than someone who needs to learn how to do something besides eat when they're stressed. This is not a contest with your co-workers to see who can lose five pounds the fastest; it is about you achieving your long-term health and fitness goals.

SELF-ESTEEM

There are a lot of issues that can affect weight, but there are also a lot of issues created by being overweight. Low self-esteem is probably the biggest obstacle to overcome. My self-esteem was incredibly low. Now, most people that know me, both now and then, would find that hard to believe. I am very friendly and outgoing and come across very secure and confident.

Little did anyone know how insecure I really was. I would laugh, joke around, and talk to just about anyone. While I did this, no one ever seemed to notice that I couldn't look them in the eye. I would always look slightly to the side of their face, or at their mouth as they spoke. Since I'm so short, it made it easy to never quite look all the way up into their eyes. If I looked into someone's eyes, I might accidentally see what they thought of me. What if they thought I was disgusting? What if they thought I was gross? What if they thought I was a joke? What if they thought I was a terrible person? What if they thought it was such a shame that I "let myself go"? It was a risk I wasn't willing to take.

I hadn't been able to look a man in the eye for about ten years, a woman in the eye for about three years, and, for the last year, I couldn't even look myself in the eye. You might think that that sounds like an exaggeration and that it isn't even physically possible, but I assure you it is possible and it is not an exaggeration. I would get ready for the day without looking at myself as a whole person. I would look at my mouth to make sure I didn't have toothpaste on my lips, look at my hair to make sure it was in place, and call it good. I could go an entire day with something on my face and never realize it because I didn't dare look at myself. Without ever having to face myself, it was easier to pretend I was still okay. You can live in a happy little place if you never have the courage to face the truth. Think happy thoughts, think happy thoughts, think happy thoughts...

As I lost weight my self-esteem started to improve. I started to have confidence in who I was. I was more secure and felt more comfortable in my own skin. I didn't feel that self-loathing and that sense of being judged by those around me. As I felt better about myself on the inside, it started to change how I interacted with people on the outside. I was finally able to look people in the eye. It was nice to have some of the confidence I had always pretended to have. I could carry on a conversation without feeling like I was a big faker. I was able to look myself in the eye. *Hi, I'm Lisa, nice to meet you. I have the strangest feeling I've met you before. Yes, I think I met you once, a long, long time ago.*

If you struggle with self-esteem issues, I encourage you to not be too hard on yourself. When you start to make yourself a priority by taking that first step towards your health and fitness goals, you validate yourself as a person, and your self-esteem will start to improve. You are an important, beautiful, and amazing person and I am so proud of you for finding the courage to take that first important step.

SELF PERCEPTION AND HOW IT AFFECTS WEIGHT

How I perceived myself definitely affected not only my weight, but my feelings about my weight. When I was young and thought of myself as a dancer, I dressed like a dancer, held myself like a dancer, and looked like a dancer. In my mind I looked the part of what I identified myself as.

When I started having children I didn't worry about how I looked, because in my mind I looked like I was supposed to: a pleasantly plump mom. That's part of being a mom, isn't it? Looking round and soft with a nice comfy lap to snuggle children in. A little fat and frumpy. Wearing "mom jeans" with the front of my shirt untucked and baby spit-up on my shoulder. Two days from my last shower and six weeks from the last time I shaved my legs. I was a mom and I looked the part.

I never once considered trying to look attractive or sexy. Homeschool moms look plain, no makeup, no fancy nail polish, no flashy accessories, hair simple, clothes comfy and frumpy. Heaven forbid I look anything but wholesome and nurturing, concerned only with the education of my offspring. Personal appearance didn't even get a passing thought on the list of priorities. I was plain, just like the image everyone thinks of when they hear "homeschool mom."

Are you starting to notice a pattern? How I identified myself in my mind was reflected by how I looked on the outside, and how I looked on the outside influenced how I identified myself. This holds true on many levels. What beliefs I had about myself that I felt were truths were reflected in how I perceived myself. A lot of my extended family had issues with weight so I *believed* that I was genetically predisposed to be fat. Most women put on weight after they have children, so I *believed* that mothers should look fat and frumpy. After two knee surgeries and back surgery, I *believed* it was impossible for me to be active and fit.

What we believe about ourselves impacts not only how we identify or perceive ourselves; it affects our perception of whether or not we think we can change. If we believe we are genetically supposed to be fat, we won't try to change. We will blame our genetics and our family tree, all while happily consuming thousands of calories and blissfully ignoring anything that even comes close to looking like exercise.

If we believe that we're supposed to look a certain way due to life factors such as having children, we won't even think about trying to change. We will just join in with everyone else when they complain about the extra weight they are carrying around post-baby and, just like everyone else, not do a single thing to change it.

If we believe that achieving health and fitness are out of our reach due to such health factors as chronic pain, injury, arthritis, diabetes, fibromyalgia, or MS, we will point to our ailment and how it limits our ability to be active or lose weight without even thinking about what we are still capable of. I know there are people who identify themselves not as a person who has a specific health issue, but as the health issue itself. They are consumed by the process and progression of their health issue to the point where they no longer see their health issue as *part* of who they are, but *who* they are.

If you use your perceptions about who you are, how you think you should look, and the factors you believe as unchangeable truths as excuses to not even try to lose weight or get healthy, you might want to start changing the way you think. If you identify yourself, as a person, by an illness or a disease process, by your life factors, or by your genetic code, you do yourself a great injustice. You limit not only how you see yourself, but what you feel you are capable of.

If you feel like no one in your family is fit or healthy you will never try to make the changes necessary to achieve health or fitness. If you feel that all women who have had children must fall victim to love handles, cellulite, and flabby bellies, you will not look for opportunities to improve your health, fitness, or appearance. If you feel your health challenges make any attempt at health and fitness something beyond your physical capabilities, you will never realize all of the things you really can do.

If, instead, you start to think of yourself as a person who can overcome challenges, someone who is successful in all they pursue, someone strong and capable, then you are well on your way to achieving the goals you set, whatever they may be.

As I lost weight, not only did my clothing size change, but the way I felt I looked in my clothes changed. My perception of how I looked changed. I remember when I lost the first 35 pounds in four short months; I felt like I was so thin. I felt like I looked amazing and I acted like I looked amazing. Yes, I was still heavy, but I wasn't as heavy as I had been, and that changed how I saw myself. That change in how I perceived myself was a huge turning point for me. I no longer felt trapped inside a body that I felt didn't accurately reflect who I really was.

I started to identify myself as someone who was fit, healthy, attractive, and sexy. I started to dress in a way that reflected how I saw myself. Gone were the "mom jeans," denim skirts, oversized sweaters, old-fashioned frumpy tops, and sensible shoes. My wardrobe took on a split personality between the two ways I saw myself. On the fit and healthy side, my wardrobe consisted of athletic shoes, yoga pants, running shorts, athletic tops, and sports bras. On the attractive and sexy side, there were cute jeans, heels, form fitting shirts, sexy little dresses, lingerie from Victoria's Secret, jewelry, and makeup. My perspective about how I looked had definitely changed.

KEEP IT IN PERSPECTIVE

Sometimes a healthy dose of perspective is all we need to turn our thinking around. I was recently having a "fat" day, and I felt like I didn't look good and was feeling out of sorts. I had to pick up a few things at the store and, while I was there, I decided to get myself some new yoga pants. As I left the store with four pairs of children's yoga pants I had to laugh at myself. Three short years ago I was shopping at a plus size store and now I'm getting my pants in the children's department. Guess my "fat" day wasn't as fat as it could have been. I needed to keep my perspective.

Now I want you to think of two women, both 5' 4", both size 16. The first woman doesn't think about her wardrobe and doesn't do her hair or makeup. She wears clothes that don't fit her well. They are sloppy, baggy, and unflattering. The epitome of fat and frumpy. The second woman spends a lot of time and effort making sure her wardrobe flatters her body. She always has her hair done and would never consider leaving her house without makeup. She is sexy and confident. The difference between these two women is not just their wardrobe; it is their self-esteem and their perception about who they are and how they look. Let's say we look closer at these two women.

The first woman was once a high school athlete who could eat anything she wanted. She stayed active in college, but her ability to eat whatever she wanted without gaining an ounce has disappeared. Fast forward fifteen years where a sedentary desk job, two children, and a diet of fast food consumed in the car while driving between her kids' after-school activities has caused her weight to slowly increase to the size she is today. She isn't sure when her weight got so high, it just sort of happened. She is embarrassed by her weight and wishes she could look like she did back in high school, but doesn't see how that is possible, so she is defeated and has given up hope.

Now let's look at the second woman. In high school she had all kinds of curves that made the boys look twice and all the other girls jealous. Over the years she has put on weight, but she feels that the added weight has only enhanced her voluptuous figure. She always dresses in a way that flatters her shape and her Saturday nights are never spent alone. She feels that she looks better now than she did when she was younger and has a long list of admirers as proof.

Both of these women are the same size, but how they perceive they look is vastly different. The first woman is self-conscious and embarrassed; she feels unattractive and uncomfortable in her own skin, with her self-esteem and confidence levels low. The second woman feels like she looks amazing; she is confident in her appearance and feels sexy and attractive, and her self-esteem and confidence levels are high.

The first woman might look just as attractive as the second woman, but she sees herself as unattractive and that clouds all of her thinking. A woman is not sexy because she is a certain size; she is sexy because she perceives herself as sexy. Her perceptions about how she looks affects her confidence and self-esteem which work together to influence how she feels about herself.

If you can honestly look at yourself and evaluate what beliefs you hold on to and who or what you identify yourself as, you can start to change those beliefs and perceptions. Instead of seeing yourself as fat and frumpy, unattractive, the victim of genetics or a health issue, or incapable of achieving health and fitness, try to see yourself as a strong, confident, capable, sexy woman who isn't afraid of any challenge. Imagine the possibilities of what you can accomplish!

HOW OTHERS PERCEIVE YOU

How others perceive you can have a big impact on how you feel about yourself. Think of those two women again. If the people around them were asked to describe them, what would they say? The first woman might be described as the typical soccer mom. End of story. Most people don't look much past the initial label they put on others. They form their opinion of what type of music somebody listens to, what type of activities they enjoy, how they spend their time, and what their personality is like based on the label they placed on them within moments of meeting them.

I remember going to events with my husband and having people's eyes glaze over when they heard I was a stay-at-home mom. They immediately mentally dismissed me as having nothing interesting or knowledgeable to say about anything that might be remotely pertinent to them. In their minds, as a stay-at-home mom I couldn't possibly discuss anything other than my children and what stage of toilet-training they were in. When I started homeschooling my children it became worse. As a homeschooler I fell outside the socially accepted norms, and the perception people have of what a homeschool mom was was even worse than what their perception of a stay-at-home mom was. As a homeschool mom, I must be some sort of religious fanatic, so people went running the other way in fear that I would try to convert them.

There's nothing like being dismissed as less interesting than a paper bag, or as some kind of weirdo, to color the way you feel about yourself. Their perceptions about you may be totally false, but that doesn't change how they treat you, and you start to believe that you are unimportant or boring or strange because that is how everyone treats you. That is how others' perceptions of you can affect how you perceive yourself.

Yet, sometimes, others' perceptions of us may be more accurate than our own perceptions. Think of someone who struggles with an eating disorder. The reflection they see in the mirror is vastly different from what the people around them see. As I lost weight, I would look at myself in the mirror and see me, but at some point it became difficult to see myself objectively.

People would look at me and say "You're so tiny!" and I kept looking at myself in the mirror trying to figure out what they were talking about. I would see how I looked, and it didn't look "tiny." Were they talking about how short I was? As more and more people would say I looked tiny, I started to think that, just maybe, it might be true.

One night, I was talking to a lady in the sauna at the gym, and she said, "I've seen you working out here; you're pretty badass." I had no idea what she was talking about. She was smiling at me when she said it, and the tone of her voice implied it was a compliment. I didn't want to look like a complete idiot by asking her what she meant, so I smiled back at her and said, "I'll tell my trainer." What I really meant was "I'll ask my trainer what you're talking about." I found out later that, yes, it was a compliment.

It was really strange when other people started to compliment me on how I looked. I wasn't expecting it at all, and I'm afraid that, at times, my response to a compliment wasn't always the socially correct one. Once, my husband and I were out on a date, and there was a young family at the restaurant whose kids were busy being kids, so the mom came up to us and apologized for her kids being loud. I told her not to worry, we had five kids so we understood. She looked at me and said, "You have five kids! You don't look like you have five kids, your legs look amazing!" Socially acceptable manners would indicate that the correct response to her statement should have been "Thank you." But I had recently reached my weight goal and was feeling pretty excited about it, and, in my excitement, I responded, "I know!" I was completely horrified that I had actually said that out loud, but the lady, who was busy looking at my legs, didn't seem to notice my social faux pas.

One of the strangest things about losing weight is that I didn't realize how different I looked to other people. To me, I just looked like me, but to other people I looked like a different person. One morning I went to the local members only warehouse store. I handed the clerk my membership card and started taking the groceries out of my cart. The clerk looked at my membership card and asked me, "Is she with you?" I looked around. I was all alone in line. I must have had an "I have no idea what you're talking about" look on my face because the clerk clarified, "Is Lisa with you?" Now I must have looked at her like she had lost her marbles. "I *am* Lisa." She looked at the picture on my membership card and looked at me with disbelief. "I'm going to have to see some I.D." I pulled out my driver's license to verify who I was and explained that I looked different because I had lost weight. She looked at me in awe and asked, "How did you do it?"

PERCEPTIONS ABOUT WHAT BEAUTY LOOKS LIKE

Sometimes the way we perceive ourselves is distorted through an outside source. Comparing ourselves to an unrealistic ideal we have in our mind can greatly impact how we feel about our weight and the way we look. We need to be realistic when we think about how we want to look or how much we want to weigh. If you have unrealistic expectations based on what you have been led to believe is beautiful or attractive, you could be setting yourself up for disappointment.

Throughout history, society and our culture often dictate what is perceived of as beautiful or attractive. Think of the paintings of those beautiful Rubenesque women: curvy, sensual, and feminine. The pin-up girls of the 1940s, showing off their curves to the delight of all the World War 2 soldiers. Marilyn Monroe and how her flirtatious confidence captured the imagination of a nation. Women who looked like women and were proud of their feminine curves were what society considered beautiful.

More recently there has been a shift in what society and culture are deeming beautiful and attractive. Starting in the 1960s, the super-thin, boyish look made popular by Twiggy became the ideal women were suddenly held to. Runway and magazine models became increasingly thinner, and the ability to count every vertebrae on a model's spine became commonplace. Some photos of what society was now dictating as beautiful and desirable looked shockingly similar to photos of holocaust victims.

As this shift in what society now viewed as beautiful took a turn from voluptuous to emaciated, women started to suffer the repercussions. Suddenly there was a market for all kinds of crazy diet fads and trends as women tried to reach that unrealistic and impossible ideal image. Not surprisingly, this is when society also became familiar with the concept of distorted body image and the horrific illnesses anorexia nervosa and bulimia. Women were suddenly going to extreme lengths to try to look a certain way they were never meant to look.

I know there are people out there who look at magazines and television and see models and actors and think that that's what they want to look like. I wonder, though; are you *sure* you want to look like that? Do you even know what that person *really* looks like? Most magazine pictures are photoshopped, and actors have professional makeup artists and hairstylists to make them look a particular way. What they look like at home when they get up in the morning is probably pretty close to how you look when you get up in the morning.

Do you really want to look like a runway model? A walking skeleton with a grumpy look on your face? A Victoria's Secret model? A walking skeleton with fake boobs? An actress who doesn't even look like herself anymore because she's gotten so much plastic surgery? All orange with a fake tan? Unable to showemotion because your face is frozen from botox? How do you *really* want to look?

Women are put under a tremendous amount of pressure from external sources to look a certain way. What a disservice the media has done to real women. The images of actresses and models, who have had face-lifts, nose jobs, lip plumping, botox injections, breast implants, butt lifts, tummy tucks, and liposuction and are then airbrushed and photoshopped to perfection, have more and more real women turning to plastic surgery to try to fit into this impossible ideal of how a woman should look.

When I started to lose weight I started to look at how other women looked. Not fake women, real women. How did real women look? How did they look in their 20's, 30's, 40's, 50's, and beyond? How do real women's bodies change as they age? Where did I fit in the spectrum of how real women looked? I talked to a lot of people and I realized something. Real men like the way real women look. Real men are not perfect and real women are not perfect, but that is the way it is supposed to be.

Not everyone is the same height, build, weight, or size. We are all different. On purpose. Wishing you could look a way that will never happen will only frustrate and discourage you. Try to look the best you possibly can for you, instead of trying to look like someone else. Be happy with the skin you're in; stop trying to make yourself look like some media-created ideal and embrace the challenge of looking as good as you can for you, no matter how you're built.

I might want to look like a Victoria's Secret model, but that will never happen. No amount of diet and exercise will suddenly make me tall and thin with long, lanky legs. I might want to look all lithe and willowy, but no matter how many weights I lift I'm not going to suddenly have smaller bones. I might want to look curvy with an hourglass shape, but there are no exercises that will make me sprout some nice, curvy hips.

I am not tall. I do not have long legs. I am not small-boned and willowy. I am not curvaceous. I am short and sturdy with broad shoulders, narrow hips, and muscular legs. I am just the way I am supposed to be. This is how I *really* look, and I refuse to apologize for looking like a real woman.

So, forget what that poor, starving, fake girl in the magazine looks like and take a look around you. Really look at how other women look and I think you will be pleasantly surprised to find that there aren't that many real women who look like the girl in the magazine. Take what you think you're supposed to look like and replace it with a healthy and fit version of what you see in the mirror. Because that, my friends, is what will soon be looking back at you.

CHAPTER THREE

FACTORS THAT AFFECT WEIGHT LOSS

<u>SUPPORT SYSTEMS</u>

It is important, when doing any type of weight loss program, that you get the support you need. Some people need constant reassurance from a person significant to them; some people need the companionship of a support group; some people need accountability from an outside source; some people need general guidelines from an online program and advice from chat groups; some people need nutritional counseling; some people need a personal trainer; some people need a structured plan that they can easily follow without having to think about it too much; some people need a friend to do it with them; some people need encouragement from someone who's been there, done that. How support works for you is an extremely personal thing, so get the support that will be the most beneficial to you.

Be aware that the type of support you need may change during your weight loss journey, or that you may need several different types of support. At first, you might not want anyone to know that you're starting your journey, so you don't have that outside pressure. Or you may want as much support as you can get. Do what works for you. Everyone's needs are different depending on their personality and where they are in their journey. Whatever support you need, don't be afraid to ask for it. You are important and your health is important.

Some people like having someone join them on their journey, some people like to travel alone. If you have a friend that needs someone to join them, but you feel more comfortable alone, don't feel obligated to do something you're uncomfortable with. Suggest another friend or a different type of support that you are willing and able to provide, and find the support you need for yourself. What works for one person may not work for another. What works at first may not work in the middle or at the end of your journey. Be flexible, and be aware of your changing needs.

I created a support network. I had people that supported me with my diet, people that supported me with exercise, and people that just supported me. Most of my support came from people I met at the gym. The gym is a great place to find people with similar goals and similar struggles. People who take their health and fitness seriously. People with a mindset similar to mine. People I could talk to about what was important to me. People who understood eating every few hours and concerns over calories and protein ratios. Having people that understood me was tremendously helpful, because sometimes I think my family thought I was crazy. Sometimes I think they were right.

After working hard to reach a weight loss goal, I had a less than healthy weekend of eating out which caused me to put back on the three pounds I had just lost. I was trying to mentally give myself a pep talk, telling myself I would get back on track and stay focused this week and the weight would come off again, when my husband noticed I was upset. He asked me how many pounds I had gained. I didn't answer him because I was still trying to mentally encourage myself, but he kept asking me to tell him how many pounds I had gained. To admit out loud that I had failed was too much for me to bear and, in my frustration, I slammed down the spoon I was cooking with and shattered my glass top stove.

Losing weight is a highly emotional process and, unless someone has done it, is in the middle of doing it, or works with people who are doing it, it is a difficult process to understand. My husband hadn't meant to upset me; he was trying to reassure me that the weight I had gained was probably due to the excessive sodium from eating out and that I would be able to lose it quickly. What he didn't understand was the significance of what he was asking me. Those three pounds for me were a huge setback. Yes, the three pounds might have been water weight from the sodium and therefore a little easier for me to lose, but they also could have been three pounds of fat and that would take me another month to lose. Unfortunately, I didn't know which category the three pounds were in and that was extremely frustrating.

My husband doesn't ask me about my weight anymore. He's afraid he'll have to buy me a new stove. Instead, if we go out, he hides the scale for a few days so I'm not upset by any temporary increase in my weight. Sometimes it is hard to know how to support someone when they are losing weight, because you're not sure what will encourage and what will offend. Try to let those around you know what is helpful and what is not so they are better able to support you on your journey. They can't read your mind, so try to let them know before you have to buy a new stove.

Getting support is vital to achieving success, and so is rewarding yourself for success. I am always quick to ask for a high-five when I do something I am proud of, or reach a new goal. I won't *ask* for the high-five; I will *tell* someone "High-five me!" My trainer immediately responds to this statement and asks for clarification later. Once I was checking in at the gym and my friend at the front desk asked me if I had reached the weight goal I had set for myself. I enthusiastically responded, "Yes!" followed with "High-five me!" Some other gym rats in line behind me had overheard our conversation, and they high-fived me as well. I will never turn down a high-five.

GOT YOUR BACK

My trainer definitely has my back. He's quick to hold me accountable, quick to reassure me, and quick to come to my defense. The gym I went to had personal trainer classes that utilized the gym for their lab. I knew they were there, but didn't really pay attention to them. That is, until the day one of the students approached me in the locker room. This student proceeded to tell me that her entire class would turn and look at me when I worked out. When she told me that, I thought I might pass out. The thought of other people looking at me while I worked out filled me with terror; the thought of an entire class looking at me made me want to die. This student then proceeded to tell me I was doing something wrong. Wait, what? I do what my trainer tells me to do, how can it be wrong?

The next day I text my trainer, 'You working today? Wanted to talk to you about personal trainer class analyzing my work out and telling me I'm doing something wrong.' Less than a minute later I got a call from my trainer. As soon as I heard his voice I just started crying. I was so distraught over the personal trainer class looking at me I just said, "Don't let them look at me. I don't want them to look at me." Needless to say, my trainer had my back. He went straight to the school and let them know that the class did not have my permission to analyze my workouts, that the exercises I was doing were correct, and that no one from the class was to ever approach me.

I was so freaked out by the thought of my workout being critiqued that for the first time in my weight loss journey I didn't want to go to the gym. *Knowing* I was being looked at while I worked out was far worse than *thinking* I was being looked at. It was my worst nightmare coming true. If the personal training class was looking at me, were other people looking at me? I scheduled a session with my trainer the next day because I felt vulnerable working out on my own and I wanted my trainer there to protect me. I have to say it was one of the hardest training sessions I ever had. I was on the verge of tears the entire time and felt like I had to throw up. My trainer was patient and encouraging and, I think, secretly hoping I wouldn't cry again.

It caused such a strain on me that it triggered a violent migraine with debilitating vertigo and nausea similar to when I first was sick. All of my new-found confidence was undermined by one person's thoughtless comments. I wanted to go to the gym, but was paralyzed with fear. My family encouraged me to go anyway. "That lady is dumb, Mom," they would tell me. While I agreed with my family on the lack of that particular person's intelligence, I couldn't bring myself to work out without the security of my trainer.

The feeling of being looked at wasn't entirely a product of my insecure, self-conscious imagination and that was extremely difficult for me to deal with mentally. I felt like everyone in the gym was not only looking at me, but critiquing me. I felt like the exercises I did were only valid if I was doing them with my trainer.

Ironically, I found comfort in the glass-walled exercise room where I would dance. Even though the walls were glass and everyone could still see me, it felt safe. No one could tell me I was dancing wrong. Dancing is a personal expression and therefore cannot be wrong. The one thing I had longed to do, but had been afraid to do, suddenly became my refuge. I would "hide" in the exercise room, the music in my ears, dancing in my safe little world.

While I continued to gain confidence I still relied heavily on my trainer for support. I didn't realize how much until I suddenly didn't have him. There was a new gym opening in town and my trainer was leaving to go to the new gym. I knew I still needed his help and so I decided to go to the new gym to continue working with him (the poor guy is never going to get rid of me).

The transition wasn't easy for me. There was going to be a four-week gap between him leaving the gym we were at and the new gym opening for business. At our last session he gave me my chart, telling me we'd pick up at the new gym. I thought I'd be fine for the four weeks, but without that accountability I was afraid. What if I blew up like a balloon?

A mutual trainer friend offered to help hold me accountable, so I wouldn't lose my focus. While it was nice to still have that accountability, it wasn't the same. My trainer and I have a great rapport and work extremely well together. My personality is very excitable and driven and my trainer is very calm and focused. A lot of my sessions include him reining me in and settling me down. I often have a mental image of me jumping around after him like a little dog yapping at his heels saying, "What are we going to do today, huh? What are we going to do?"

As the four weeks came to a close I was anxious to get back on track. Opening day arrived and I was excited. We'd show all the people at the new gym what a real training session looked like. I showed up at the gym ready to go. It was so crowded you could hardly move, wall-to-wall people, loud, chaotic, stressful. All of the people made me extremely nervous. The newness of the facility made me nervous. The change made me nervous. It was like going to the gym for the first time, and I was totally uncomfortable. I tried to do what I would normally do before a training session, a ten-minute warm-up on the elliptical and some stretching. My heart was racing and I felt sick to my stomach. I was overwhelmed by all of the people and felt lost and out of place. That is not how a gym rat should feel. I tried to calm down and get it together before my session, but I couldn't. My trainer came looking for me when I didn't show up at the trainer's desk. He found me sitting on the floor trying to "hide" in plain sight.

As soon as I saw him I just started to cry. I told him I couldn't do it. There were too many people, and it was too much for me to deal with. I wanted the security of a gym I knew and was comfortable with. I wanted my "home" gym. I wanted the safety of people I knew around me. Just like my first session after the personal training class critique, this session was terribly difficult for me. It is hard to focus and lift weights when you're trying to deal with years of emotions regarding self-image, self-esteem, and self-consciousness.

The trooper that he is, my trainer took it in stride. He calmed me down, reassured me I was okay, and made me feel better. Those first weeks at the new gym were very hard on me. I couldn't swim or dance there, and only went for my weekly session with my trainer. For all of my other workouts I went to the gym I had started at. The gym that felt like home, the gym with all of my friends.

I had created a gym "family" that I was comfortable with at my first gym. I knew most of the staff and recognized a lot of the other gym rats. I could spend 30 minutes just chatting before I even started my workout. The new gym intimidated me. I didn't know where anything was. I didn't know where I fit in. I didn't have the security of all my friends, and I didn't like it.

The new gym was offering a conditioning class for teens three times a week, so I signed up one of my kids. Since I was already there, I figured I might as well do my workout. So I started to learn my way around and started making a new support system. I'm not sure when the new gym started to feel like home and the staff like family. It was a gradual process. I can't be entirely positive, and I know he'd deny it, but I'm pretty sure my trainer smirked with satisfaction when I started to dance and swim at the new gym.

SABOTEURS

When you lose weight or try to improve your overall health and fitness, there is a chance you might run into a saboteur. A saboteur can be anyone: your mother, your spouse, your best friend, or a co-worker.

Change makes people uncomfortable, even when it's a change for the better. A lot of people feel threatened when someone close to them starts to lose weight. Sometimes they feel guilty, like they should lose weight too. Sometimes they're afraid that the person losing weight won't love them if they're not thin as well. Sometimes they're worried; are you going to make them eat healthy also? Sometimes they're unsure. They just don't know where they fit in anymore. And sometimes they're just downright jealous.

A saboteur can sabotage you knowingly or unknowingly. For example, if you have always been a "good eater" and suddenly you're making different food choices, your mother might unknowingly sabotage you by offering you your favorites when you're visiting. She might even feel hurt that you're not eating what she has prepared for you, in turn making you feel guilty. Your mother is not knowingly trying to sabotage your healthy eating choices; she is just doing what she's always done.

It could be your friend, spouse, or co-worker who wants to have lunch with you or go have a few drinks. They want to continue doing the activities they have always done with you and they don't understand why you don't want to do them, too. Once again, this change in your eating pattern and lifestyle choices may cause hurt feelings in your friend, spouse, or co-worker with resulting guilt on your end.

The best thing to do with this type of unknowing saboteur is to let the person know what you are trying to do and ask for their help. If your mother/spouse/friend/co-worker understands what is happening and feels like they are part of your team, they can go from unknowing saboteur to amazing asset. Maybe your mom will start to find healthy recipes for you. Maybe your co-worker will go for a walk with you at lunch instead of going to a restaurant. Maybe your spouse can take you on a date that isn't food related. Maybe your friend will go to the gym with you, and maybe you could be the inspiration they need to start their own journey.

Sometimes, unfortunately, the sabotage isn't unknowing. Sometimes your saboteur knows exactly what they're doing. This type of saboteur is typically motivated by jealousy. They may make rude comments and try to belittle your efforts. They may flaunt less healthy food choices in your face. They may come right out and say that you will fail. They may insult you or try to mentally or emotionally hurt you. If you have this type of saboteur it is best to limit or eliminate your interaction with them if at all possible. It is naive to think that you may not encounter this type of sabotage, so be prepared.

Do not let this type of saboteur inside your head. They do not have Jedi mind powers that will work on you. You are much too strong to let them have any type of power over you. Remember that this person is motivated by jealousy. They are jealous of *you*. They are jealous of your will-power, jealous of your ability to succeed at a goal you have set before yourself, jealous of the way you look (because you look *amazing!*), jealous of the attention you are getting because of your weight loss. The journey you are on is difficult and you need to surround yourself with support, not saboteurs.

CHANGING ROLES

My support system has changed as I've gone through this journey, and my role within the support system has also changed. Now I give support instead of just receiving it. People on their journey look to me for advice, input, moral support, a shoulder to cry on, practical tips, inspiration, encouragement, reassurance, high fives, a pat on the back, compassion, and empathy.

It took awhile for me to get used to the idea of being someone whom others looked to for nutrition, health, fitness, and lifestyle advice. Who I am to tell someone what to do? Then I realized I had more credibility to those around me than some celebrity touting the latest diet trend. I was a *real* person, who *really* lost weight. I was right in front of them. They could see how I *really* looked. Living proof that weight loss is possible for "regular" people and that you're never too old to get in shape and achieve your health and fitness goals.

Unlike a lot of people interested in health and fitness, I have been on the other side. Some doctors, dieticians, and trainers have never had trouble with their weight or struggled to learn how to eat and exercise. I can understand your feelings of insecurity, embarrassment, and fatigue. I know what it's like to feel overwhelmed and not know where to begin. I know how scary it is to think about changing everything you know and are comfortable with. I know what it's like to fear failure.

I also know what it feels like to need a smaller pair of jeans. I know how it feels to look at yourself in the mirror and like what you see for a change. I know how it feels to have the energy to do everything you want to do. I know how it feels to accomplish a goal you set for yourself. I know that you would love to know these things, too.

I love talking to people at the gym and encouraging them on their journey. I love being able to impact people in a positive manner. I love watching others succeed in meeting their goals. The gift of health is the best gift of all, and I love telling others how they can achieve it.

GOAL SETTING

There are many goals you can have on your journey toward health and fitness. You can have activity goals: I want to be able to walk a mile. You can have body image goals: I want to look fit and healthy. You can have endurance goals: I want to have energy all day long. You can have size goals: I want to fit in last year's jeans. You can have weight goals: I want to weigh a certain weight. You can have fitness goals: I want to improve my cardiovascular strength. You can have health goals: I want to lower my blood pressure. Just as you have your own journey to health, you have your own goals.

I was constantly setting new goals on my journey. New weight goals, body image goals, endurance goals, self-esteem goals, and fitness goals. I was always striving toward something new. I need a goal to keep me focused. My mom once asked me, "Isn't maintaining a goal?" My emphatic response was "No!" Maintaining is a lifestyle, not a goal.

Goals are a great way to determine success and a great way to define what it is you really want to achieve on your journey. You may realize that, for you, being able to have energy is your main goal. Or, you may find out that deep down you have always wanted to run a 5k or triathlon. Setting goals helps you determine the focus of your journey.

Goals are both short term and long term. Your long-term goal may be to lose 20 pounds, your short-term goal may be to lose one pound this week. You may have a long-term goal of looking fit and healthy, and a short-term goal of being able to see your feet. Short-term goals help you reach your long-term goal.

Once you have reached one goal, it is time to set another goal. Let's say your first long-term goal is to be able to walk a mile. Your short-term goal might be walking around the block, then two blocks, etc., until you reach your goal of walking a mile. Once you can walk a mile you might want to set a new long-term goal regarding your weight, then maybe a body image goal, and so on. Setting new goals will keep you motivated and focused.

When you reach a goal you need to reward yourself. No, that does not mean eating chocolate chip cookies as a reward for losing five pounds. Reward yourself with some new scented candles, a bubble bath, some perfume, high fives from your support system, some new workout shorts, a victory dance, a massage, some new earrings, a pedicure, some new workout music for your iPod, or some new jeans (in a smaller size).

FITNESS REWARD

I'm pretty sure that I am probably one of a very small group of very strange people who reward their fitness goals with exercise. If I do my extreme intervals, I will reward myself by swimming. If I get all of my workouts in, I will reward myself by dancing. I use the exercise that I like as a reward for completing workouts, and that is pretty strange.

GOAL WEIGHT , BMI, AND IDEAL WEIGHT

What is the difference between goal weight and ideal weight? Depending on your goal weight, there may not be much of a difference at all, or they could be worlds apart. Goal weight is the weight that you would like to weigh, ideal weight is the weight that is ideal for your body and is sometimes referred to as your "natural weight." Contrary to popular opinion, the BMI (body mass index) is not necessarily the same as ideal weight.

Consider a body-builder with muscles on top of muscles. With all of that lean muscle and very little body fat, they most certainly do not appear to be overweight, unless you look at the BMI chart. Some of these super-fit athletes fall into the obese category. "How can that be?" you may ask. Easy. The BMI chart is not based on body fat (which is a better indicator of overall health and fitness); it is only based on height to weight ratios.

When I started out, I set my goal weight at 130 pounds. I felt that it was a realistic goal that I could achieve. While I hadn't weighed myself since I hit the 180-pound mark, I was pretty sure I was close to 190 pounds. For me to get back down to 130 meant I needed to lose about 60 pounds. I knew it would be hard, but I was up for the challenge.

My trainer told me that I could do better than 130 pounds. He challenged me to do 129 pounds so that I would exceed my goal. The day I hit 129 pounds my trainer and I strutted around the gym saying "129!" and showing people my fat picture and taking all the high fives we could get. It was an amazing feeling.

Once I hit that goal I was really excited, until I compared my weight to the BMI chart. The goal weight I had worked so hard to reach had me soundly in the "overweight" category. I was so disappointed. I was in excellent shape cardiovascularly and did not look overweight, but that was not reflected by the BMI chart.

My victory of hitting my weight goal was no longer a victory in my mind. If I would have gone in for a physical or applied for life insurance I would have been classified as "overweight." I was frustrated and upset that all of my hard work didn't seem to matter. So I decided to set a new weight goal.

Still, my goal weight and my ideal weight were not the same. Now, you may be thinking that my ideal weight was even lower and harder to get to, but you're wrong. Once I hit my final goal weight of 115 pounds I decided I could ease up on how strict I was with my eating plan and workouts. My weight settled into a four-pound weight fluctuation between 118-122 pounds, which is a normal fluctuation for healthy individuals. It led me to realize that, even though my goal weight was 115 pounds, my ideal or "natural" weight was approximately 120 pounds.

Even though my ideal weight was heavier than my goal weight and at 120 pounds I was pushing the upper limits of what is considered "normal or healthy" BMI, I finally listened to my trainer and stopped obsessing about what the scale said (Shhh! Don't tell him I actually listened to him, it will go to his head). I focused on other aspects of health and fitness, like how I looked and felt.

When setting a goal weight it is important to set realistic goals based on age, gender, body frame size, and body fat percentages, not just what the BMI chart tells you you should weigh. Your goal weight may change as your weight loss journey progresses. You may adjust it higher or lower depending on how you lose fat and gain muscle.

DON'T GET HORMONAL ON ME

Signing up for training sessions at my new gym, I had an interesting conversation with the gym manager. I was asking how the personal training packages were priced, and he proceeded to tell me that you pre-order your training sessions based on how much weight you want to lose. If you wanted to lose 20 pounds, based on the average weight loss of 1 to 2 pounds per week, you would purchase 10-20 weeks of training. My response was, "Who loses weight like that? Dudes?" While the manager was contemplating how to respond to my question, I emphatically voiced my opinion. "Dudes suck. Women don't lose weight like that. It's so unfair."

While it's true I started out losing weight at that rate, that is not how I continued to lose weight. The closer I got to my goal, the harder it was. The first 35 pounds came off at the one to one and a half pounds per week, then I plateau-ed for eight weeks, then the next 15 pounds came off at 3/4 to 1 pound per week. The last 15 pounds were an agonizing one-step-forward, two-steps-back process that was directly related to my menstrual cycle.

Hormones were definitely affecting my weight loss. I had a one-week window during each menstrual cycle in which I could lose weight. It was extremely difficult to see my weight loss goal be so close and yet so far. It was like running a race and, as soon as I saw the finish line, instead of sprinting to the end I had to crawl.

During my one week to lose weight I had to be super vigilant on my eating plan and I pushed myself extra hard at the gym. I had to make the most of my opportunity while I could. I guess I could have just been content with where I was at with my weight, but I had set a goal and I wanted to reach it.

Every so often my trainer would ask me, "How's your weight?" Sometimes I'd give him a number, sometimes I'd just say, "Good." Sometimes I'd say, "It sucks to be a girl." It's true that hormones play a role in weight loss and weight gain, and sometimes being a girl does suck. I would bemoan the fact that women have higher body fat percentages than men and how unfair it was that men could lose weight easier than women. Unfortunately, all my complaining didn't change the fact that my weight loss was hormone related. I had to work with my body instead of fighting it. My hormones didn't keep me from reaching my weight loss goals; they just made me take the scenic route on my journey. The day I met my goal weight still felt amazing, even if it took longer than I had hoped. All of my hard work had finally paid off with a number on the scale that matched the number I had set my heart on.

While I was losing weight my trainer kept telling me, "People see inches, not pounds." It's not like we're walking around with our weight over our heads in flashing lights. Thank God! So even though the scale didn't move as quickly as I wanted for those last 15 pounds, my body was still changing quite a bit.

I often hear people say, "Muscle weighs more than fat," and that reminds me of a riddle my kids used to ask me when they were little. "What weighs more, a pound of feathers or a pound of bricks?" they would giggle as they would try to trip me up. I would pretend not to know the answer and they would laugh hysterically as they delivered the answer: "They weigh the same!"

A pound of muscle weighs the same as a pound of fat. However, the volume of a pound of muscle is way different than the volume of a pound of fat. Think of a lean 16-ounce steak and a 16-ounce bag of marshmallows. Now, which one looks better in your jeans? People see inches, not pounds, so if you're lean and muscular you may look way better than someone who weighs the same but is made out of marshmallows.

Try not to focus too much on the scale. Instead, really look at yourself. Evaluate how you look in your clothes and how your clothes fit you. If your hormones are slowing down what the scale says, but you need to buy smaller jeans, then you're doing fine.

STRESS AND SLEEP

Stress is a major factor that can impact weight loss. You can be eating healthy and working out regularly but still not lose weight if your stress levels are too high. So, how do you get your stress level to a manageable point? Good question.

If you're dealing with short-term stressful situations you could try one (or more) of these options.

1. Go to another room where you can't see or hear the stressful situation.

2. Close your eyes and take some deep, cleansing breaths while consciously relaxing your neck, shoulders, and back.

3. Use some aromatherapy oils; any scent that you find soothing will do.

4. Take a relaxing bath or soak in a hot tub.

5. Sit in a sauna or steam room.

6. Take a brisk walk around the block.

If you're dealing with a more constant form of stress like caring for an elderly parent, a high stress job, marital difficulties, etc., you may want to add in some other strategies to help you with your stress levels.

1. Yoga.

2. Meditation or prayer.

3. A relaxing massage.

4. Acupuncture.

5. Support group.

One thing people tend to overlook is the healing power of a good night's rest. Your body needs rest, just like it needs food and exercise. If you're working out and pushing your body without giving it the rest it needs to recover, you're not going to get very far.

It's okay to need sleep. That is when your muscles recover from a workout and your brain gets the rest it needs to function properly. Some people see getting eight hours of sleep as laziness or weakness. Not true! You are neither lazy nor weak if you listen to your body and give it the rest it needs. Without proper rest your body is going to burn out. So go ahead and get forty winks; you'll thank yourself in the morning.

CHAPTER FOUR

GRADUAL DIETARY CHANGE

GOTTA EAT

Eating is probably the most crucial part of achieving success when following a weight loss regimen. When I started out, I would do great following my healthy eating plan during the week, but would always blow it on the weekends. All of the good I did during the week was totally undone by the bad. It wasn't until I got serious and took care of my diet *every day* that I started to lose weight. For me, taking care of my diet means I eat every 2 - 3 hours, I eat a lot of protein, I eat high-fiber complex carbohydrates, I eat lots of fruit and veggies, I eat low fat or fat free dairy, I watch my sodium intake, and I drink at least eight glasses of water every day.

Before I even started to lose weight, I understood enough about myself to know that I couldn't eat simple carbohydrates for breakfast. If I didn't eat anything for breakfast I did better than if I ate a sugary bowl of cereal for breakfast. With simple carbohydrates I would be jittery and starving within the hour.

So, when I started to try to eat healthier I figured I'd start with breakfast. It's the most important meal of the day, right? I knew I couldn't eat sugary cereal for breakfast, so what's a healthy breakfast food? Let me think...healthy breakfast food, healthy breakfast food, healthy breakfast food... Of course! Yogurt is healthy and it has protein. Okay, what else? Fiber. Fiber is good for you and there are tons of high fiber cereals and high fiber bars. Fruit is good; it's natural and healthy. There we go, my healthy breakfast: non-fat yogurt, high fiber bar, and a banana. Done.

So that's what my beginning steps into healthful eating looked like. It wasn't crazy or drastic or hard to do. I started doing something I thought I could do. Let's say I had been reading some weird nutritional/diet book that told me I needed to eat fermented tofu, lima beans, and brussel sprouts every day. I wouldn't have done it. Period. It's unappealing on so many levels and so far removed from what I would normally eat that it would never work. I changed my diet gradually over time, "cleaning" it up over weeks and months, because that was easier to do.

GRADUAL DIETARY CHANGE

What is gradual dietary change? It's exactly what it sounds like: changing your diet gradually over time to increase your chances of being able to maintain the changes and achieve long-term success. Do you ever hear someone say, "I'm doing this thing where I eat real food every couple of hours"? Probably not. How many times have you heard someone say, "I tried low-carb for a few weeks," or "I tried the cabbage diet, once," or "I did the juicing and raw food diet for about a week"? Probably a lot. People say they did it or tried it; no one says they're doing it long term because they're not realistic eating plans. They are so different from what the average American is used to eating that they are hard to stick to.

Most people are too tired or stressed out to think about overhauling their diet. Creating a meal plan, grocery shopping, cooking, and planning ahead aren't at the top of most people's list of "fun things I want to do this weekend." Thinking about all of the work involved with making a major dietary change is exhausting to most people. We live in a society that doesn't slow down. Every day people are rushing here, rushing there, with a "to-do" list a mile long that they never seem to get to the bottom of. Constant demands on time and energy leave most people too tired to do anything but try to survive the week and re-group on the weekends.

People don't want to have to stop and think about what they should be eating; they want someone to take the guesswork out of it for them, because it's too hard to try to figure out on their own. When I was heavy, if I looked at a book or magazine that said it had this "miracle diet," I would more often than not just look at the menu options to see if what they suggested for meals was something I would like to try. I wasn't really interested in their nutritional theory; I just wanted to know what to eat. I think a lot of people are the same.

While people like to have their meals laid out for them so all they have to do is follow, it can still seem overwhelming. The meal plan doesn't tell them *how* to do it. It just says, "Eat this." So most people look at the meal plan and don't know where to start. They tell themselves they'll try it next week when they have time to figure it out. It is so different from what they're used to that it scares a lot of people. "How can I eat like that? I don't have time to prepare all those different meals. What is the rest of my family supposed to eat?"

I was talking to a lady at the gym one day, and she asked me, "Did you have to change the way you eat?" She asked it with such an expression of unwillingness to change that I answered "yes" as gently as I could. I could tell by her demeanor and body language that the idea of changing her diet seemed to be such a difficult and overwhelming challenge that it bordered on impossible.

I wanted to explain to her that she could gradually change her diet so that her chance of success with a new healthy eating plan would increase, but her next question totally threw me off. "What do you eat, *salad*?" The way she said "*salad*" was as if she was asking me, "What do you eat, *poop*?" I felt bad for her and her obvious dismay at the prospect of eating said "*salad*," but she needed the truth. "Yes, I do eat salad." She looked so disappointed when I gave her the answer that she didn't want to hear.

It seems to me that a lot of the people I talk to want to be thin, but no one wants to go through the process of losing weight. Losing weight is hard; it takes a lot of effort. It is scary and intimidating and seems impossible. The likelihood of failure is enough to deter most people before they even start. There are literally thousands of diet books out there that can give all kinds of strategies for losing weight, yet even with guidance from a book, weight loss is a daunting task.

That is why I advocate gradual dietary change. It is easier to maintain one or two dietary changes at a time than a complete dietary overhaul. It feels less restrictive and doesn't seem as hard. You eat an elephant one bite at a time...with your *salad*.

Now, in our "instant" society, gradual change is looked upon as a thing of the past. People want to lose weight *now*. The question is, do you want to lose weight now, or do you want to lose weight forever?

Sometimes the cost of the "healthy" food is a big deterrent. To those people who claim that healthy food isn't more expensive than junk food, I say, that's a big, fat lie. Healthy food *is* more expensive. A bag of chips is way cheaper than a container of organic mixed baby greens, so which one is going to end up on your plate? White bread, processed lunch meat, and cheese food product is way cheaper than whole wheat bread, sliced chicken breast, and real chunk cheese. Which one is going on your sandwich? Boxed macaroni and cheese is way more affordable (and easier) than making whole wheat pasta with sautéed chicken breast and fresh vegetables drizzled with extra virgin olive oil; what will make it to your table at the end of a busy day? If you're like the average person, it probably depends on the state of your budget.

Here's the good news. While the healthy food is more expensive up front, it nourishes your body better. You won't have to keep trying to eat to give your body what it wants and needs, because you already did it. Think about it. You can eat an entire family size bag of chips with your sandwich of white bread, processed lunch meat, and cheese food product and still feel hungry enough to go for the box of cookies afterward. Then at dinner, your boxed macaroni and cheese, as the main entree without vegetables and protein, doesn't give you what you need so you eat two or three platefuls and follow that with your favorite television-watching snack.

Let's say that instead of eating the cheaper, less healthy options you have the whole wheat bread with chicken breast and real cheese, and a salad of mixed greens. You won't need that bag of chips or the box of cookies, because you won't be hungry. Then, when you go to eat your dinner of whole wheat pasta, chicken breast, and vegetables, you're not starving (for once) so you eat one serving and put the rest in a container for tomorrow's lunch and skip the late night snack. You can see how this eventually works out so your budget can stay on track. What doesn't work is buying both the healthy and less healthy options; that can double your grocery bill.

You can change one or two things in your diet for a week or two, then maybe change something else for a few more weeks, then tweak it a little bit in a month, and so on. Over the course of 3-6 months you could totally overhaul your diet without feeling overly deprived or restricted. The gradual change will be easier to handle mentally and emotionally, it will be easier to manage financially, and it will be easier to stick to long term.

What if I told you that, by gradually changing your diet, you won't feel as drained at the end of the day? That by nourishing your body throughout the day instead of starving it or trying to fill it with empty calories, you won't feel like you're going to collapse by the time you go to bed? What if I told you that gradually changing your diet will help you lose weight and give you more energy? Would you be willing to try? Come on, you know you want to.

RESTRICTIVE DIETS

You can jump right into eating like how I eat now and you'll probably lose weight. Will you keep it off? Hard to say. When we, as human beings, feel like we're being deprived of something we will rebound by over-eating at the first opportunity. It's human nature; you can't avoid it. You might think you have lots of self-control and that it wouldn't happen to you, but if you restrict too quickly and too severely you're going to binge.

WHAT DO YOU MEAN LETTUCE IS A CARB?

When people hear the word "carb" they think of bread, pasta, rice, crackers, and cereal. They think carbs are starches. There are three basic categories of food: proteins, carbohydrates, and fats. So, if it isn't a protein or a fat, it's a carb. All fruits and veggies are carbs, including lettuce. When you hear people talking about not eating carbs what they usually mean is they aren't eating starches. Restricting an entire food group is not only dangerous, it is extremely difficult. It would be impossible to eliminate all carbs from your diet, unless you're a lion.

Restrictive diets that exclude entire food groups are nearly impossible to maintain long-term and are therefore doomed from the start. Yes, it sounds easy. "Just eliminate carbs from your diet and you'll lose weight," and that *will* result in weight loss, but only temporarily. When you deprive your body of the essential nutrients it needs, your body starts to starve and it won't function properly. Your body will start to demand what it needs, and that is when the restrictive diet fails. All of the nutritional needs your body has for the energy from complex carbohydrates will need to be met, and you will put back on all of the weight you just lost, and maybe a few more pounds on top of it.

I had to go on an extremely restricted diet due to some trouble with Candida overgrowth. I could only eat rice and quinoa for starches; eggs, beef, chicken and fish for protein; and select low-sugar veggies for nutrients and fiber. I tried to cheat and eat yogurt, oatmeal, and coffee while restricting all of the other foods, but that didn't work. Sigh. So I gave up the yogurt, coffee, and oatmeal and finally started to feel better.

After 11 long weeks with no fruit, dairy, bread, etc., I went a little crazy and started to eat things I would never have eaten before I went on the Candida diet. Things like candy and cake. Yummy! I made things like french toast with syrup and grilled cheese sandwiches. So good! I totally loaded up on fruit: grapes, bananas, watermelon, cantaloupe, honeydew, mango, nectarines, strawberries, blueberries, raspberries, and blackberries. Yes, I bought all of these fruits at one time and proceeded to eat pounds of fruit every day. Each bite of fruit was like a little bit of heaven, a holy experience accompanied by choirs of angels singing. Of course, my weight went up when I started eating all of the restricted foods again, but I had the knowledge and tools I needed to get back on track.

Most people just give up and go back to eating the way they're used to when they get off-track on their eating plan, because they feel like they've failed and their "regular" diet is easy and familiar to them. Just because you make some food choices that might not be the best, it doesn't mean you should give up on a healthy eating plan and go back to eating whatever you feel like. It means you enjoyed some food that you were missing, but now you need to re-focus.

If you just need to lose a few pounds for an upcoming wedding, reunion, Christmas party, etc., then a short-term, restrictive diet overhaul may work perfectly fine for you. Maybe not. What happens when you go to the wedding, looking fabulous after dropping those 5 pounds, and you drink like a fish and indulge in every scrumptious-looking morsel that passes by? You deserve it, you worked hard to fit into that dress, and you need some "real" food after eating so healthfully the last couple weeks. Now that the goal has been reached (you fit in the dress you wanted to wear), you can go back to eating how you normally eat. How do you look and feel after a week back on your "regular" diet?

Maybe you feel tired and sluggish. Maybe you feel bloated and uncomfortable. Maybe you feel downright gross. Maybe you wish you looked as good as you did when you slipped that sexy little dress on. But you know you can't stick to the restrictive diet without going crazy. So what do you do? Let me think. Let me think. I know the answer, just give me a minute. It's on the tip of my tongue. Oh! Now I remember: gradual dietary change. Where have I heard that before?

REAL LIFE EATING

Now if you think I eat one hundred percent healthy one hundred percent of the time, you would be one hundred percent wrong. I eat as healthfully as I can, but I'm still human. I have a crazy busy schedule just like everyone else, so I understand how easy and convenient fast food is and I do eat there occasionally. I like to go out to restaurants when I'm on a date with my husband, and sometimes a girl just has to have her chocolate. I tell you this so you realize that eating healthy is an overall pattern of how you eat, not one specific meal.

For example, when I was heavy, my overall eating pattern consisted of fast food several times a week, junk food every day, and lots (and I mean lots) of high fat, high calorie food I would prepare at home. Now, my overall eating pattern consists of healthy food choices daily, with eating out 2-4 times a month. When I eat out now, it looks a lot different than it did when I was heavy. Fast food before was typically two large burgers or crispy (deep-fried) chicken sandwiches, fries, soda, and sometimes ice cream; now it is grilled chicken (no mayo) and a side salad (mustard, not salad dressing) with my water.

For those of you that are scared to give up all of the food that you love, let me assure you that you can still eat the things you love. You just need to learn how to enjoy them in a way that fits in with your eating plan. Instead of eating half a pepperoni pizza with a 2-liter bottle of soda in front of the TV right before you go to bed, you can eat two slices of a chicken and veggie pizza with a salad for lunch after your workout. You still get the pizza, but you get it in a more appropriate serving size, with the added nutrition of the salad, and you eat it at a time that is more conducive to losing weight.

When I eat now, I am very aware of not only what I am eating, but how what I'm eating will affect both my weight and my health. If I know I'm going out to dinner with my husband in the evening I have to be very careful with my eating the entire day so I can enjoy the meal. This does not mean I don't eat all day; it means I am very careful with how much fat, sodium, and starchy carbs I eat.

Restaurant food tends to be high in fat and sodium, and most restaurants almost always include some sort of starchy carbohydrate either with the entree or as a bread basket, and that is why I am careful not to consume too much of these things earlier in the day. I also know that when I go out to dinner with my husband I will be eating later than I normally do and that, combined with the higher fat, sodium, and calorie content, can affect my weight.

IT'S BETTER THAN FRENCH FRIES

A lot of people tend to get caught up in all kinds of ridiculous nit-picking when it comes to making healthy food choices. They get all crazy over things, like if you eat fruit or vegetables out of season they don't have as many nutrients, or what kind of lettuce you should eat, saying this one has more nutrients and is therefore healthier, blah, blah, blah. I answer that with the statement I always tell myself when I eat something that maybe wasn't the best option. "It's better than french fries." I tell myself that to help me remember to keep it in perspective, because maybe I shouldn't have eaten the full fat ranch dressing with my carrot sticks, but guess what? It's better than french fries.

When I found out I was pregnant with my surprise sixth baby, there was some serious comfort food on the menu. At that point in my journey I had already reached my weight goal and had developed a new relationship with food. When I ate the comfort food I was consciously deciding to eat it, not just responding to the stress of a surprise pregnancy by eating.

As I sat in a fast food restaurant letting some of the kids play while my daughter and I discussed the new baby over french fries and ice cream, I knew exactly what I was doing. I was choosing to ignore my healthy eating plan as I mentally tried to wrap my brain around the fact that I was going to have another baby. As we were leaving the restaurant, I started to say my mantra of "It's better than french fries," but then I stopped when I realized that, oh no! that *was* french fries.

That had always been my culinary measuring stick, which helped me keep things in dietary perspective, and now I had gone ahead and eaten them. As I stood there, not knowing what to say, my daughter laughed, gave me a hug, and said, "Don't worry, Mom, it will be okay." And you know what? She was right. It *was* okay.

When I ate something that didn't fall into the "healthy" category, the world didn't stop turning on its axis, the stock market didn't crash, the sun didn't fall from the sky, there wasn't an earthquake, and there wasn't a news flash on the 6:00 News about me eating something I shouldn't. My dietary indiscretion was just a blip on the dietary radar. Yes, eating french fries wasn't the healthiest choice I could make, but one poor decision did not make me a bad person or an unhealthy person; it made me a regular person.

CHAPTER FIVE

EATING PATTERNS

DIFFERENT EATING STYLES

As I have gone through my weight loss journey, I have talked to a lot of people and have discovered that there are different styles of eaters. You may have never thought that eating can have a particular style, but it does. Your particular style of eating will influence how you need to approach your weight loss. Weight loss is an extremely personal journey that is influenced by many factors, and diets that have a one-size-fits-all approach can set you up for failure. When you're aware of your eating style it is easier to understand how you need to change your eating habits.

Just as every individual is unique, so is their eating style. I have identified five different styles of eaters, but I'm sure there are a lot more. Try to honestly evaluate how you eat in relation to the following categories.

STARVERS

These are the people who go all day without eating, except for coffee or soda. The constant stress and/or busyness of the day keeps their mind off of food. They don't get any calories when they need them and try to make up for it at the end of the day by consuming their entire day's worth of caloric needs, and sometimes more, in one sitting right before bed. Which, unfortunately, doesn't work the best.

These are the eaters that have stopped listening to their bodies. Their body might be sending them hunger signals, but they have learned to ignore what their body is saying. They may notice that they feel a little hungry, but the deadline for their project is making a bigger impact in their brain. It's like when you're a kid and your mother tells you to do something. You hear her voice, but what she is saying doesn't register in your brain.

After a while, your body says again that it's hungry and yet again it doesn't quite register fully in your brain. This is like when your mom is telling you, "This is the second time I'm asking you to do this." You hear her say this statement but you can't remember what it is she told you to do in the first place, so you figure it must not be too important.

Now your body is starting to get upset by your lack of response to its hunger signals, so it sends a very clear message to you that it needs food. This is when you might get a headache, feel nauseous or lightheaded, or feel completely exhausted and be unable to focus. Instead of stopping for twenty minutes to eat so you feel better, your hunger signals make you feel more stressed about all the things you still need to do even though you're not feeling well. You grab a cup of coffee, hoping that will help you focus, and you keep going because you feel a tremendous time pressure. This is when your mom is getting frustrated at your lack of response and starting to get in your face. She has raised her voice and is letting you know that you'd better do what she has told you to do. You're almost done doing whatever it is you're doing, so even though you know you need to listen to her, you figure you'll do it just as soon as you're done.

This is the final straw; your body has had enough of you ignoring it all day. It is telling you that you need to feed it *right now.* You finally realize that you haven't eaten all day and you feel like you're starving. You figure you'd better eat something quick or you're going to pass out from hunger. You grab some fast food and eat quickly to make up for not eating all day. You eat so quickly that your body can't send full signals to your brain and, even if it did, you're so used to tuning out what your body tells you that you don't listen. And you eat thousands of calories to make up for not eating all day. This is the point where your mom is now yelling at you and you quickly go do what she has been telling you to do all day. She is upset and angry with you and doesn't understand why she had to yell at you to get you to respond. You think your mom is crazy; you did what she wanted and you can't understand why she is so upset. This type of eater really needs to learn how to listen to its mother, er, body.

EMPTY CALORIE EATERS

Perhaps you're like a lot of other people who munch down on three doughnuts that someone brought in to share at work for breakfast. Then hurriedly eat lunch at a fast food restaurant, washing it down with plenty of soda, making sure they re-fill their cup so they have something to drink with their two snack size bags of chips and the package of cookies for their mid-afternoon snack. After a long day at work, they don't feel like cooking so they pick up something to eat on the way home. For a treat, they have half a carton of ice cream while they watch their favorite TV show and fall asleep on the couch watching the news.

These people are trying to listen to their bodies and feed it throughout the day. Unfortunately, they're choosing the wrong things. Your body needs calories, energy, and fiber from complex carbohydrates. It needs the muscle building power of protein. It needs the vitamins and nutrients from vegetables and fruits. It needs bone-building calcium from dairy. It needs essential fatty acids, and it needs plenty of water.

Let's say your body needs calories and energy, so it tells you, "I'm hungry; could you give me something to eat?" You respond by having a cup of coffee or a can of soda and a candy bar. Your body didn't need caffeine, sugar, or chocolate, so it says, "Hey! I'm still hungry; could you get me something to eat?" So now you respond by having a bag of chips. Your body didn't want fat and sodium. It wanted energy from complex carbohydrates and protein, and it's getting angry that you're not giving it what it wants. "Hey! I'm serious; give me something to eat *right now*." So you run and grab a slice of pizza. Refined carbohydrates with just a touch of protein from the cheese is still not sufficient and not what your body needed. Now your body has had enough. It wants complex carbohydrates, protein, some nutrient-packed fresh vegetables, and some healthy fats. "Come on! Where's the food? Don't you hear me saying I'm hungry?" That's when you grab your fast food dinner on the way home and fill your body up with empty calories, sodium, and fat, with nary a vegetable in sight. Your body is tired now. It's been telling you all day what it needed, but never got.

If your car needs gas, you don't put air in the tires. You don't change the oil. You don't buy a new battery. You take it to the gas station and put gas in the tank. That's what you need to do for your body. When it needs good nutrients and calories, feed it what it needs.

ACCIDENTAL EATERS

This is the group of people that gets "accidental" calories without even realizing it. How? Very easily. You make your kids lunch. You lick the extra mayo off your finger between sandwiches. Then you take one or two chips from each child's plate. Then you make your lunch. After lunch you clean up, eating the last few bites the kids left because "good food shouldn't go to waste." You have just consumed two meals worth of calories without realizing it. If someone were to ask you, you just had a sandwich and a few chips because you didn't even realize you ate all that extra food.

Sometimes you're cooking dinner and can "accidentally" consume almost an entire meal's worth of calories. Tasting for seasoning, popping some of that chicken in your mouth when you're cutting it up, checking to see if the pasta's done, trying out that new salad dressing, eating a piece of the french bread while you're slicing it for dinner, licking the spoon and/or bowl when preparing dessert. You weren't eating; you were making dinner. And you just "accidentally" consumed 500 calories.

Maybe you work in an office where people always bring food to share, or have a bowl of candy on their desk. You have a nibble here and a nibble there without tasting it because you're distracted by the project you're working on, so it doesn't register in your mind that you're eating. All of these "accidental" calories add up. Quickly.

I remember once I was putting on more weight and I couldn't figure out why. I was talking to a friend about it and they asked if I had changed my diet in any way. I said no, I was still eating the same. Then I suddenly realized that a Krispy Kreme doughnut shop had opened in town, and I would get a couple dozen every week when I was on that side of town and snack on the doughnuts with the kids. Here I was, eating at least a half dozen doughnuts every week, and it didn't even register in my brain until I was talking to someone else about it.

This type of distracted eater can eat an entire family size bag of chips throughout the day without realizing it because they grab a handful here and a handful there. They are often in denial about what and how much they eat. They may prepare a healthy breakfast, lunch, and dinner and think they are eating healthy all while conveniently forgetting they ate an entire box of cookies, a bag of beef jerky, half a bag of chocolate chips, and a six pack of soda.

They tend to only see the calories they eat when they sit down to eat, and easily forget any calories they have consumed outside of the dining room table. Their conscience might prick them once in awhile, trying to remind them of everything they really ate throughout the day. They will put their fingers in their ears and say, "What's that? La, la, la, can't hear you," and keep pretending to themselves and everyone around them that they are eating in a healthy manner.

OVER-EATERS

The over-eater is what their mother might refer to as a "good eater." A hearty appetite used to be considered a good thing. "Picky eaters" were frowned upon and you were expected to clean your plate. You might have been praised for eating so well and given dessert for eating all of your food.

This type of eater is often a people pleaser who associates cleaning their plate with praise for a job well done. This type of eater will often eat even when full because, if someone offers them something to eat, they feel it would be rude to refuse. When the other person seems happy with their response it justifies the feeling that they should eat whatever is offered to them.

The over-eater style of eating can start with the "good eater" mentality or it can be a form of stress eating or emotional eating. If you're under a lot of stress or dealing with difficult emotions and you turn to food for comfort, you can quickly compound the stress or emotional eating problem with an overeating problem. You might think if one cookie makes you feel better then two cookies will make you feel twice as good and the entire box of cookies will make everything bad go away. Unfortunately, once you wake up from the sugar coma everything comes back.

It is important to recognize which category of over-eater you fall into. The emotional and mental aspects of losing weight will be different for the "good eater" over-eater and the stress/emotional over-eater.

THE FOODIE

This type of eater is the one that really enjoys food. Pouring over recipes and cookbooks, watching cooking programs on television, trying new foods, recipes, and restaurants. This type of eater is usually an excellent cook or someone who really knows the difference between good food and great food. The foodie has no trouble finding time to eat. Any time is the right time to eat. The foodie is always up for trying a new culinary experience and they tend to "live to eat."

The foodie will tell you about a trip they took by telling you about the restaurants they went to and the food they ate, not the sights they saw. They might say something like, "We went to Disneyland, and they had the best little ice creams shaped like Mickey Mouse ears," or "The Grand Canyon was great; they had the cutest little restaurant just outside the park," or "The Renaissance Festival was so much fun, I ate way too much."

The foodie will research food and restaurants on the internet, reading restaurant reviews, recipe reviews, and food blogs. They may refer to famous chefs as if they know them. "Mario made the most amazing pasta I ever saw." They may have an impressive cookbook library or huge files of recipes from the internet. The foodie can spend hours thinking about food, building recipes and menus, watching cooking programs to learn new techniques and recipes, and experimenting in the kitchen.

The foodie doesn't think twice about going out of their way to find great food. A restaurant 30 miles away, or driving for an hour to get to a gourmet food store to find some obscure food item they're interested in trying isn't out of the question. Spending three weeks planning a menu and two days in the kitchen preparing for a dinner party is a joy for them.

The foodie loves all things food related. The foodie usually understands a lot about flavor profiles and how to build amazing meals. They know what they like to eat and really enjoy eating it. They are culinary adventurers who aren't afraid to try new things. They usually have a well-stocked pantry with lots of ingredients the average person may not have even heard of. The foodie definitely knows food.

CHAPTER SIX

EATING STRATEGIES

EATING PLANS

Now, I know some of you have skipped to this chapter to see what it's all about without having to read the entire book. I can't blame you for that; it's what I would have done when I was learning how to get healthy. Getting started with a healthy eating plan can be very intimidating and stressful, which is why I advocate gradual dietary change. Gradually changing your eating habits is a manageable way to incorporate healthy eating patterns for lifelong success. Sounds good, doesn't it? So, how does it work and how do you get started?

First, you should identify what type of eater you are, so you know where to start. If you can't readily determine what type of eater you are, keep a food journal for a few days and that should give you the information you need to get started. If you seem to fall somewhere between two different types of eating patterns, choose whatever feels like it will work better for you. Once you have determined what type of eater you are, you can follow the gradual dietary change eating plan that best suits your specific needs.

This is a personal journey where you determine the speed at which you travel. I can't tell you when you'll be ready for the next step. That is totally up to you. What I can do is show you the next step so when you're ready you know where to go. You might want to try one thing at a time for short periods of time before moving to the next step, or you may want to try a couple at a time for longer periods of time. You might start with longer adjustment periods and gradually decrease the amount of time between dietary changes, or start with short adjustment periods that get longer the further you get into the process. Whatever feels the most comfortable for you is what will work for you and your long-term goals. Remember, this is a process that takes time. If you feel panicky about the next step, then you're not ready. Don't beat yourself up if you feel like it's taking too long. You're trying to undo years' worth of unhealthy eating habits.

STARVERS

1. Start with breakfast.

2. Increase water intake.

3. Eat lunch.

4. Healthy dinner.

5. Healthy snacks.

1. Start with breakfast. For those of you who are not used to eating more than once a day, the recommendation to eat 5-6 small meals a day (which is the best for you and your health) may seem an impossible task. For this group of people I suggest starting with a portable, drinkable breakfast. Breakfast really is the most important meal of the day, so if you can start there you are headed for success.

Now, you might be saying to yourself, "I can't eat first thing in the morning, it makes me nauseous," or "I can't eat breakfast, my mornings are so crazy I'm lucky I can get out the door." I will make this as painless as possible. Make yourself a power-cino or other protein shake (see recipes) before you go to bed and it will be ready for you in the morning. Since most starvers only drink coffee or soda during the day, the power-cino is a good start. It is something you drink, but with the added nutrition of protein powder. This is your first step towards health.

2. Increase water intake. Starvers tend to have a caffeine addiction whether they realize it or not. Caffeine in and of itself is not necessarily a bad thing, but if you're drinking all of that caffeine you're probably not drinking water also. The lack of water, combined with the diuretic properties of caffeine, means you are probably in a perpetual state of dehydration. Proper hydration is vital to your overall health. This doesn't mean you can't ever have caffeine-containing beverages, it means you need to increase your consumption of water. Try replacing a cup of coffee or can of soda with a bottle of water, gradually decreasing your coffee/soda intake and increasing your water intake. Weaning yourself off of caffeine may take a while, so don't hesitate to make some other dietary changes during this process if you feel you're ready.

3. Eat lunch. Once you start having something to eat for breakfast, you might start to get hungry for lunch. This is a good thing! It means your metabolism is starting to wake up. If you are still uncomfortable with cooking, meal planning, and eating, you could have another protein shake for lunch. Do not have more than two protein shakes a day. You need to learn how to eat, not continue in your "starver" eating pattern. If, at this point, you feel ready to eat a real meal for lunch, then go ahead and add in a healthy lunch option.

4. Healthy dinner. Now you need to take a look at your dinner. If you feel that you can't possibly avoid fast food or eating out due to your schedule or your lack of culinary skills, don't panic. This is where the gradual part really comes in handy. Start small and make changes when you feel you're ready. If all you feel like you can manage is not having dessert, then pass on dessert. If you feel like you can eat a healthier option at a restaurant, then do that. All fast food restaurants have their nutrition facts available either online or in the store so you can check out them before you order.

If you feel like you want to try to start making healthy food at home you can do that gradually too. If you normally cook like Paula Deen, don't despair! You can still make great tasting meals that you can enjoy without all of the extra calories and fat. You can start switching from less healthy options to healthier options as you feel ready for them. Try fruit or yogurt for dessert, change white rice to brown, substitute whole wheat pasta or bread for white, dress veggies with olive oil instead of butter, and have more veggies and less refined carbs.

5. Healthy snacks. Adding snacks into your eating plan will help you keep your metabolism on track. Once you add in snacks you can cut back on some of the calories you consume for your main meals. There are lots of snack options out there, so finding something you enjoy eating shouldn't be too difficult. By the time you have added in your snacks you will have gone from a "starver" to a 5-6 small meals a day metabolic powerhouse. See, now that wasn't so bad, was it?

EMPTY CALORIE EATERS

1. Substitute low-fat/reduced calorie versions of snacks.

2. Increase water intake.

3. Start with breakfast.

4. Add fruits and veggies.

5. Healthy lunch.

6. Nutritious dinner.

1. Substitute low-fat/reduced calorie versions of snacks. Empty calorie eaters are accustomed to eating throughout the day, but they are often junk food junkies. They consume high amounts of calories, fat, sugar, and sodium from highly processed foods. The empty calorie eater tends to be someone who isn't entirely comfortable in a kitchen or may not know how to cook at all.

For you, I recommend starting with some baby steps. You're not going to need to break a sweat thinking about breaking out the pots and pans or eating celery sticks all day. You're going to start choosing healthier versions of what you already eat. Most companies offer low-calorie or low-fat versions of their products, so start there. Eat the baked chips instead of the fried ones, the low-fat cookies instead of the regular version, frozen yogurt instead of ice cream.

You need to stay aware of your portions. When you substitute the lower fat or lower calorie versions for the real deal that doesn't mean you get to eat more of them. If what you're eating has 50% fewer calories, you don't eat 50% more. Try to get the single serving option instead of the "family size." Eating an entire "family size" bag of baked potato chips kind of defeats the purpose.

2. Increase water intake. After you have "cleaned up" your snacks a bit, you should add some water to your snack. Eating a low-calorie portion-controlled snack may leave you feeling hungry, so have a glass of water with it. Think of the water as part of your snack. For your mid-morning snack, have your baked chips *and* water. For your afternoon snack, have low-fat cookies *and* water.

3. Start with breakfast. Now we're going to healthy up your breakfast. Start your day off right and it will be easier to stay motivated to stick with your eating plan. A protein smoothie in the morning is a great way to start. It is quick and easy and requires no cooking. If you prefer to start your day with a bowl of cereal, try a healthier cereal whose main ingredient isn't sugar or high fructose corn syrup.

4. Add fruits and veggies. With your healthy start to the day and your better choice of snack foods, you're getting to the part where you need to increase your fruits and veggies. The easiest way to do that is to add fruits and veggies to your snacks. Have your low-calorie treat *and* water *and* a fruit or vegetable, gradually replacing your processed snacks with fruits, veggies, and a protein.

5. Healthy lunch. Let's look at your lunch now. You may eat lunch at a restaurant every day due to work or time demands or because you just don't cook. Once again, you're going to start small. Research the nutrition facts of restaurants you normally eat at and see where you can make improvements in your choices. Replace the crispy fried chicken with grilled chicken, eat the salad instead of fries, and pass on dessert, bread baskets, chips and salsa, and soda.

If you find it difficult to make healthier choices while eating out, start thinking about making your lunch at home and bringing it with you. Avoiding the restaurant might be easier than trying to make healthy choices when you see and smell all of the other less healthy options. It might take awhile to change your eating habits, but hang in there. You can do it!

6. Nutritious dinner. For the empty calorie-eater/junk food junkie, eating a nutritious dinner means making a nutritious dinner. This may be the hardest part for you. The kitchen may be a room you are completely uncomfortable with and the thought of cooking makes you break into a cold sweat. Don't panic! I'm here for you. Just as you've done through this whole process you're going to start small.

You can have dinner in fifteen minutes without having to cut a veggie or take out a pot or pan. There are lots of foods out there that you can prepare with minimal time, effort, and cooking skills. You can take a chicken breast, lean steak, or frozen fish fillet (not breaded or processed) and put it on a George Foreman Grill with some seasoning of your choice, and steam some broccoli, green beans, or vegetable blend in the microwave and put a pre-cut salad in a bowl.

You did it! You went from an empty calorie eater who didn't know how to fill their tank with gas to a smart and savvy healthy eater running on all four cylinders.

ACCIDENTAL EATERS, OVER-EATERS, AND FOODIES

1. Be aware.

2. Lighten up.

3. Drink more water.

4. Just say no.

5. Divide and conquer.

1. Be aware. I've placed the accidental calorie eaters, over-eaters, and foodies together because the underlying issue they all need to deal with is awareness. The accidental calorie eater isn't aware of everything they are eating, the over-eater isn't aware of what normal portions look like, and the foodie isn't aware of how many calories are in what they're consuming.

For these eaters, the first step will be a reality check. If you fall into one of these categories you're going to have to keep a food journal. Now, when I was heavy the thought of writing down everything I ate was horrifying. I knew I ate too much and I didn't want to put it in writing, but keeping track of my food is now second nature.

I know you probably don't want to do it, but you have to write down *everything* you eat. This isn't for the sake of making you feel bad about what you eat, it's about making you *aware* of how you eat. You can keep a food journal on the computer, you can keep track of your food using an app on your smartphone, or you can just write it down in a notebook. Whatever is easiest for you. The important thing is to do it.

Once you are aware of how you eat, you can change how you eat. When you start your food journal you become aware of your eating patterns. You can see if you tend to eat more in the afternoon or in the evening. You can see if you eat when you are stressed or bored. And you can see which situations cause you to eat more.

Now that you know how you eat, let's start to change it. Try to interrupt eating binges, accidental situations, and over-eating by trying a few of these simple tricks. Chew gum; you can't eat if you already have something in your mouth. Brush your teeth as soon as you're done eating to signal to your brain that you're done. Take your plate to the sink as soon as you're done eating and then either brush your teeth or chew some gum so you don't accidentally eat off the serving plate or your kid's plates. Don't eat on the run or eat out of the package. Sit down and pay attention to what you are eating.

2. Lighten up. Now you need to lighten up your food intake. Look at the food you eat, I mean really look. Look at the nutrition facts of what you're eating and the serving size. If you read the nutrition facts on a label without paying attention to the serving size you can get yourself into a lot of trouble. People tend to think of the package of what they're eating as the serving size and that's not how it works.

If you get a bowl of cereal, what you pour into the bowl is the portion, not the serving size. Some cereals' serving size is only 1/2 cup. Now compare that to the two cups you just poured into the bowl. Some companies will market their product saying "Only 100 calories per serving!" but their package contains two and a half servings. So you eat the entire package thinking it's only 100 calories and it's really 250 calories.

Pay attention to the food labels and be aware of serving size. Sometimes you can lighten up your caloric intake just by eating the serving size instead of your normal portion. I know it sounds like a lot of work, but start slowly and you will succeed.

For the over-eater, the real serving size may seem like you will starve to death if that's all you eat. If your normal portion is four serving sizes then, by all means, do not abruptly reduce your portion to the actual serving size. If you try to lighten up too quickly you will feel hungry and deprived and that is when most eating plans fail. To succeed you will need to gradually reduce how many servings you eat.

It is important to be completely honest with yourself during this process. Pretending you always eat just one serving does not help you. Pretending you normally eat four servings when you really eat six doesn't help you. Don't feel embarrassed or ashamed when you realize how much you really eat. Knowledge is power! Take your new-found knowledge of how much you eat and challenge yourself to gradually reduce it. Take your time. Remember you are undoing years of poor eating habits.

Replace one unhealthy thing at a time. Instead of a bowl of candy at your desk, keep healthier options like cut-up fruit or vegetables, low-fat yogurt, nuts and seeds. Now, slow down and really focus on what you're eating. Don't just shove food in your mouth without really tasting it; savor what you are eating. When you slow down your eating it gives your brain and your stomach time to realize when you're full. By tweaking just a few things you can make a big difference.

3. Drink more water. Now it's time to start drinking. Water, that is. Drinking enough water is vital to your overall health, and can help curb your appetite. Sometimes you think you're hungry when really you're just thirsty. So if you feel like you want something to eat, try drinking a glass of water first. Then, if you're still hungry, eat a sensible snack. Try to drink at least eight glasses of water a day. I know this sounds like a lot and, for the foodie, it sounds completely tasteless and boring. I have some simple strategies to help with increasing water consumption in the "General Guidelines for Healthy Eating" section.

4. Just say no. Now it's time to learn to say no. Say no to the food you think is going to help you feel better. Say no to that extra serving of your favorite food. Say no to the candy jar at your desk. Say no to the new restaurant down the street. Say no to watching hours of cooking shows on television. Say no to mindless eating. Say no to obsessing about food. Say no to living to eat.

One day a friend of mine was visiting and, as she looked at the macaroni and cheese I had made for my kids' lunch, she asked me, "How can you have all this food around you and not eat it?" I hadn't really thought about it before, but it came down to me just saying no. At some point I had to take responsibility for my eating habits, and I needed to have the ability to say no.

This is where your determination comes into play. You have decided to become healthy and your food choices need to start reflecting that decision. Trust me, I know how hard this is. I promise it will get easier, and I can honestly say that nothing tastes better than success.

5. Divide and conquer. Now it is time to divide what you eat into 5-6 small meals a day. For the foodie who loves to cook, this task may be pleasant. Focus on creating healthy sensible meals that have correct serving sizes. Eating healthy doesn't mean you have to sacrifice taste, so have fun re-creating healthier versions of family favorites. Make your food pretty; enjoy it with your eyes as well as your mouth. If it looks like it tastes delicious, it probably *is* delicious.

Try to eat every 2-3 hours so you don't get tempted to overeat because you're too hungry. Watch your portions to make sure you're eating the correct serving size. You made it! You've gone from a food addict who lived to eat to someone who eats to live.

GENERAL GUIDELINES FOR HEALTHY EATING

1. Drink it up.

2. Eat the rainbow.

3. Eat like a hobbit.

4. Keep it simple.

5. Wrap it up.

1. Drink it up. I cannot say emphatically enough how important it is to stay hydrated. Drinking water will help you tremendously. Water will help you flush away fat, literally. Pun totally intended. Drinking eight glasses of water a day may sound unappetizing and really difficult to do, so here are a few helpful strategies.

You can get a 2-quart pitcher and pour your water out of it to easily keep track of your water consumption. Or you can get yourself a nice reusable water bottle and keep track of how many times you refill it. You can try using a straw if that helps you drink more water. You can measure out 8 ounces of water and try to sip it throughout an hour, and refill it every hour. Challenge yourself to drink more water every day and before you know it drinking eight glasses a day will be part of your routine.

Now, I agree that drinking plain water can get boring, but don't get tempted to add a sugar-free powdered flavor mix to your water. These products will try to tell you that it's perfectly fine to add them to your water and that it makes drinking water easier, but don't be fooled. As soon as you add something like that to your water, you are no longer drinking water. Think about it. If you add lemonade powder to your water, you're drinking lemonade, even if it's sugar free.

Instead of being tempted by all of those powdered flavors, try something real. Add a slice of lemon, lime, or orange to your water. Use a few frozen berries instead of ice. Or try my absolute favorite, a few slices of cucumber and a sprig of mint. Delicious! Drinking water doesn't have to be boring or tasteless. Get creative and make up some flavor combinations that appeal to you. You're only limited by your imagination.

2. Eat the rainbow. When you get your creative culinary juices flowing you can start experimenting with all kinds of new fruits and vegetables. Not everyone likes the same thing, so if your best friend doesn't like something it doesn't mean you won't like it. Try something new, or try mixing things you normally wouldn't, like fresh fruit in a salad or on top of your chicken. If you don't like boiled cauliflower (not sure if *anyone* likes boiled cauliflower) try roasting it in the oven instead, or eat it raw with a low-fat dip. Eat a wide variety of fruits and vegetables. Try incorporating as many fruits and vegetables into your diet as you can. They are a great way to nourish your body.

3. Eat like a hobbit. This is a reference to the hobbits in "The Lord of the Rings" trilogy, where they wanted to stop their journey so they could have something to eat. Their leader said they had already eaten breakfast and therefore would not be stopping to eat. The hobbits responded, "What about second breakfast? Elevensies? Luncheons? Afternoon tea? Supper? What about those?" Those hobbits sure know how to eat. Make sure you eat 5-6 times a day to keep your metabolism running at optimum efficiency. The better your metabolism runs, the more calories you will burn. You need to eat to lose weight, not starve yourself to lose weight. So enjoy your healthy, sensible 5-6 small meals a day and you will reap the many metabolic rewards.

4. Keep it simple. Keep your dinner simple. By this I mean you shouldn't be making huge 5 course meals for dinner. If you've eaten sensibly throughout the day you shouldn't need too much for dinner. Food is fuel for your body; you need fuel to do everything in your busy day. By dinnertime most people are winding down for the night and therefore will not need as much food (fuel). So, for dinner a lean protein paired with a salad or some vegetables should be sufficient for you. This is the only time I'm going to tell you to avoid starches (pasta, potatoes, rice, bread etc.); the energy these foods provide is not needed at dinnertime. You do not need a lot of calories for energy to sleep, so enjoy your starches at breakfast or lunch and keep your dinner simple.

5. Wrap it up. Finally, do not eat after dinner. This is prime snacking time for most people. They will unwind after a busy day with their favorite snack. This is a habit that *must* be broken. Filling up your body with a bunch of empty calories right before you go to sleep is going to sabotage all of the good choices you've made all day. If you have eaten well all day and nourished your body correctly you shouldn't need to eat after dinner; you're just used to eating after dinner. If you're missing your favorite snack, eat it before you go to the gym instead of eating it before you go to sleep.

If you can follow these simple strategies, your journey towards your health and fitness goals will be successful.

CHAPTER SEVEN

HELPFUL HINTS
AND
SAMPLE MENUS

<u>HELPFUL HINTS FOR HEALTHY EATING</u>

- Always plan ahead. Take a small, insulated lunch sack and fill it with a protein shake, cut-up fruits and veggies, yogurt, hard boiled eggs, string cheese, sandwich, etc.

- Replace high-fat, high-sugar condiments like mayonnaise or mayonnaise substitute with fat-free plain or Greek yogurt or mustard.

- Replace salad dressings with mustard, balsamic vinegar, lemon or lime juice. Make your own dressing with fat-free yogurt by adding your favorite herbs/seasonings (watch sodium content) and thin with water or lemon juice.

- Replace high-calorie, high-sugar BBQ sauces with balsamic vinegar and/or liquid smoke flavoring.

- If you can't give up your high-calorie condiments and salad dressings, try watering them down a bit. You still get the flavor, but will use much less. Don't forget to measure out your serving size.

- Try to eat as "clean" as possible (i.e. processed foods = bad). Use cooked, sliced chicken breast instead of lunch meat.

- Try to eat 5-6 small meals a day. It may seem like a lot to get used to, but try to break up your calories and consume smaller meals more frequently. Try not to get too hungry; it will make you overeat at your next meal.

- Replace all refined flours, breads, pastas, cereals with whole wheat or whole grain. Read labels carefully; some companies mislead. The ingredients should read 100% whole wheat or 100% whole grain.

- If you're eating out, look at the menu online before you go, if you can. Decide what you're going to eat ahead of time so you're not swayed by what other people eat.

- When eating out at a restaurant with very large portion sizes, ask for a "to-go" container at the beginning of the meal. When your food arrives, you can portion it right away so you don't accidentally overeat, and then you have another meal ready for another day.

- Don't be afraid to special order your meal at a restaurant. Ask for no salt or butter on your veggies, no seasoning on your meat, no cheese or croutons on your salad, lemon or Tabasco on your salad instead of dressing, and "no, thank you" when they offer the bread basket or complimentary chips and salsa.

- Try not to eat too close to bedtime. If you're really hungry, eat straight protein, egg whites, cooked chicken, or cottage cheese.

- Try to eat a protein with your carbs. Don't eat a piece of toast for breakfast unless you're having egg whites with it.

- Cook once a week and freeze meals. I cook brown rice and chicken or roast, and put them with some frozen veggies (don't need to thaw, just throw them in frozen) in a reusable container.

- Try to eat raw, not canned, veggies and fruits. The more natural the food, the more nutrients. Frozen veggies and fruits are fine as long as they don't have added sugar/sodium/fat.

- Try to avoid artificial anything.

- Don't let others make you feel bad for making healthy choices: "It's only once a year," or "Just this once won't hurt," or even worse, "Just run an extra 10 minutes on the treadmill" (as if 10 minutes on the treadmill works off an 850-calorie piece of cheesecake). Treat it like a food allergy; bad food makes you feel bad.

- Treat yourself to something you really like once in awhile so you don't feel deprived. Just limit it to the one thing you really want and eat only one measured portion.

BAD FOOD THAT SEEMS HEALTHY

- Granola-Some varieties are high in fat and calories.

- Tortilla Wraps- High in calories and often made with refined flours and high-fat dressings.

- Fruit Juice- High in sugar and calories and low in fiber.

- Vegetable Juices- High in sodium and low in fiber.

- Diet Soda- Fake everything.

- Pre-packaged "diet food"- High in sodium, highly processed, and low in taste.

- Sugar-Free Products- Artificial sweeteners are not a healthy choice.

- Restaurant Salads- Often loaded with cheese, croutons, deep-fried chicken, and high fat dressing.

GOOD FOOD THAT GETS A BAD RAP

- Eggs- Good source of protein and omega-3's.

- Dairy- Good source of protein and calcium; just keep it low-fat or fat-free.

- Avocado- High in potassium and omega-3's.

FOODS THAT CAN BE GOOD OR BAD

- Nuts and Nut Butters- Good source of protein but high in fat, don't over-indulge.

- Turkey Alternatives to Red Meat- Good source of protein, but some varieties have as much or more fat than the red meat they are replacing. Read labels carefully.

- Yogurt- Good source of protein and calcium, but some varieties have artificial sweeteners.

BREAKFAST IDEAS

Please note that all recipes can be found in Chapter Ten.

- Breakfast Banana Split (see recipe)

- Breakfast Parfait (see recipe)

- Scrambled Eggs (3 whites and 1 whole egg); one slice low - calorie whole grain bread topped with 1 t. grass-fed butter or heart-healthy substitute; ½ c. fruit

- Scrambled Eggs (3 whites and 1 whole egg) with spinach, onion, and halved grape tomatoes; one slice low-calorie whole grain bread topped with 1 t. grass-fed butter or heart-healthy substitute

- Scrambled eggs (3 whites and 1 whole egg); one slice low-calorie whole grain bread with 1 t. grass-fed butter or heart-healthy substitute; mixed salad greens dressed with 1 t. olive oil and the juice from ½ orange or lemon

- Old-fashioned oatmeal with agave, cinnamon, and vanilla extract with ½ c. frozen blueberries (defrosted) or ½ banana; 3 egg whites scrambled

- 2-3 oz. breakfast steak; one egg cooked with non-stick spray; one slice of low-calorie whole grain bread topped with 1 t. grass-fed butter or heart-healthy substitute; ½ c. berries or melon

- Brown rice with 3 scrambled egg whites; mixed salad greens dressed with 1 t. olive oil and the juice of ½ an orange or lemon

- Brown rice mixed with 1 c. fruit; 3 egg whites scrambled

- French toast made with 2 slices low-calorie whole grain bread dipped in one whole egg mixed with 2 T. skim milk; topped with fruit, yogurt, or unsweetened applesauce

- Egg Sandwich (see recipe); ½ c. fruit

- Protein cookie; skim milk or low-fat yogurt

- Protein Shake

- ½ Protein Shake; fiber bar

LUNCH IDEAS

- Turkey Burger Salad (see recipe); whole grain Crackers

- Chicken Salad Sandwich (see recipe); 1 c. sliced cucumber

- Tuna Salad Sandwich (see recipe); 1 c. veggies

- Chicken breast or lean steak; ½ c. brown rice; stir-fry blend veggies; Asian Salad (see recipe)

- Mixed greens with diced cucumber, tomato, avocado, and fresh dill topped with low-sodium tuna dressed with mustard; whole grain crackers

- Grilled chicken breast; small sweet potato with 2 t. grass-fed butter or heart-healthy substitute; mixed greens dressed with lemon juice; ½ c. unsweetened applesauce

- Grilled chicken; ½ c. quinoa; grilled or sauteed zucchini; ½ c. strawberries

- Chicken Pasta Salad (see recipe); ½ c. melon

- Sliced grilled chicken breast on low-calorie whole grain bread with 1 T. hummus, sliced cucumber, and sprouts; celery sticks; ½ c. fruit

- Grilled chicken breast on a low-calorie whole grain bun with 1 T. avocado spread (see recipe), lettuce, and tomato; celery sticks; ½ c. grapes

- Grilled tilapia on a low-calorie whole grain bun with mustard, lettuce, and tomato; ½ c. vinaigrette coleslaw (see recipe); ½ c. melon

- Turkey or veggie burger on a low-calorie whole grain bun with ketchup, mustard, lettuce, and tomato; carrot and celery sticks

- Tortilla Pizza (see recipe); salad dressed with lemon juice

- Anything on the breakfast ideas list

DINNER IDEAS

- Turkey Burger Salad (see recipe); 1 c. mixed frozen fruit (defrosted)

- Grilled steak; Garlic Green Beans (see recipe); salad dressed with lemon juice; ½ c. fruit

- Steak Salad (see recipe); Strawberry "Ice Cream" (see recipe)

- Grilled salmon; Asian Salad (see recipe); ½ c. blueberries with cinnamon and a splash of skim milk

- Grilled salmon; steamed broccoli; sliced tomato; ½ c. mandarin oranges

- Grilled tilapia; fresh herb salad dressed with olive oil and vinegar; glazed carrots; ½ c. unsweetened applesauce

- Grilled tilapia; Cucumber and Tomato Salad (see recipe); Strawberry "Ice Cream" (see recipe)

- Southwest Chicken Salad (see recipe); "Baked" Apple (see recipe)

- Lemon Garlic Chicken (see recipe); spinach salad dressed with olive oil and lemon juice; ½ c. peaches

- Apricot Chicken (see recipe); spinach salad dressed with olive oil and balsamic vinegar; ½ c. mixed frozen fruit defrosted

- Balsamic Glazed Chicken (see recipe); spinach salad dressed with olive oil and lemon juice; ½ c. mandarin oranges

- Italian Chicken (see recipe); blueberries with cinnamon and a splash of skim milk

- Pork loin; sauteed spinach and tomatoes; "Baked" Apple (see recipe)

- Roasted chicken and veggies; "Baked" Apple (see recipe)

SNACK IDEAS

- Light string cheese and fruit

- Light string cheese and veggies

- Hard boiled egg and fruit

- Hard boiled egg and veggies

- Protein bar

- Protein cookie

- Protein shake

- Cottage cheese and yogurt

- Cottage cheese and fruit

- Cottage cheese and veggies

- Yogurt and whole grain crackers

- Yogurt and fruit

- Yogurt and veggies

- High protein cereal with skim milk

- High protein cereal with yogurt

- Low-calorie whole grain bread with 1 T. nut butter, ½ c. skim milk

- Carrot, celery, or apple with 2 T. nut butter

- Almonds and fruit

- Almonds and veggies

SAMPLE MENUS

Sample Menu One

Breakfast: Oatmeal with ½ banana; 3 egg whites scrambled

Snack: Hard boiled egg; ½ banana

Lunch: Chicken Salad Sandwich (see recipe); 1 c. sliced cucumber

Snack: ½ c. cottage cheese mixed with ½ c. yogurt

Snack (optional): Celery sticks with 2 T. nut butter

Dinner: Grilled steak; Garlic Green Beans (see recipe); salad dressed with olive oil and balsamic vinegar; ½ c. unsweetened applesauce

Sample Menu Two

Breakfast: Omelette (3 whites and 1 whole egg, topped with 1 T. low-fat cheese); mixed greens dressed with olive oil and orange or lemon juice

Snack: Yogurt and 1 c. strawberries

Lunch: Grilled tilapia on a low-calorie whole wheat bun with mustard, lettuce, and tomato; ½ c. Vinaigrette Coleslaw (see recipe); ½ c. melon

Snack: Cottage cheese and carrot sticks

Snack (optional): Protein Cookie (see recipe)

Dinner: Balsamic Glazed Chicken (see recipe); Spinach Salad (see recipe); mandarin oranges

Sample Menu Three

Breakfast: Egg Sandwich (see recipe); 1 c. melon

Snack: Protein Cookie (see recipe); celery sticks

Lunch: Tortilla Pizza (see recipe); salad greens dressed with olive oil and vinegar

Snack: Cottage cheese and carrot sticks

Snack (optional): Hard boiled egg and small apple

Dinner: Turkey Burger Salad (see recipe); 1 c. frozen tropical fruit defrosted

Sample Menu Four

Breakfast: Breakfast Banana Split (see recipe)

Snack: Light string cheese and veggies of choice

Lunch: Grilled chicken; small white or sweet potato with 2 t. grass-fed butter or heart healthy substitute; mixed greens dressed with lemon juice; ½ c. unsweetened applesauce

Snack: Hard boiled egg and ½ banana

Snack (optional): Almonds and veggies of choice

Dinner: Southwest Chicken Salad (see recipe); "Baked" Apple (see recipe)

Sample Menu Five

Breakfast: 3 egg whites and 1 whole egg scrambled with 1 c. spinach, 2 T. diced onion, and ¼ c. halved grape tomatoes; one slice low-calorie whole grain bread, toasted with 1 t. grass-fed butter or heart-healthy substitute

Snack: 1 c. high protein cereal and ½ c. yogurt

Lunch: Chicken Pasta Salad (see recipe); ½ c. melon

Snack: Protein Shake (see recipe)

Snack (optional): Light string cheese and cucumber slices

Dinner: Grilled salmon; Asian Salad (see recipe); ½ c. blueberries (optional: sprinkle with cinnamon and add a splash of skim milk)

Sample Menu Six

Breakfast: Protein Shake

Snack: High protein cereal and yogurt

Lunch: Grilled turkey burger on a low-calorie whole wheat bun with ketchup, mustard, lettuce, and tomato; carrot and celery sticks

Snack: Light string cheese and bell pepper strips

Snack (optional): Almonds and small apple

Dinner: Lemon Garlic Chicken (see recipe); Spinach Salad (see recipe); ½ c. sliced peaches

Sample Menu Seven

Breakfast: 3 egg whites and 1 whole egg scrambled; 1 slice low-calorie whole grain bread, toasted with 1 t. grass-fed butter or heart-healthy substitute; ½ c. fruit

Snack: Cottage cheese and celery sticks

Lunch: Tuna Salad Sandwich (see recipe); 1 c. broccoli

Snack: Protein Shake

Snack (optional): Light string cheese and multigrain crackers

Dinner: Pork loin; Sauteed Spinach and Tomatoes; "Baked" Apple (see recipe)

Sample Menu Eight

Breakfast: ½ Protein Shake; Fiber bar

Snack: Cottage cheese and veggies of choice

Lunch: Sliced grilled chicken breast on low-calorie whole grain bread with 1 T. hummus, sliced cucumber and sprouts; ½ c. grapes

Snack: ½ Protein Shake and multigrain Crackers

Snack (optional): Hard boiled egg and veggies of choice

Dinner: Sweet & Spicy Chicken (see recipe); sauteed zucchini; Spinach Salad (see recipe); ½ c. frozen blueberries defrosted (optional: sprinkle with cinnamon and add a splash of skim milk)

Sample Menu Nine

Breakfast: Breakfast Rice (see recipe); 3 egg whites scrambled

Snack: High protein cereal; yogurt; veggies of choice

Lunch: ½ c. quinoa, sauteed chicken and zucchini; ½ c. grapes

Snack: Cottage cheese and veggies of choice

Snack (optional): Protein Shake and veggies of choice

Dinner: Grilled tilapia; Cucumber & Tomato Salad (see recipe); Strawberry "Ice Cream" (see recipe)

Sample Menu Ten

Breakfast: French toast made with 2 slices low-calorie whole grain bread dipped in one whole egg mixed with 2 T. skim milk; topped with ¼ c. cottage cheese and ¼ c. yogurt mixed; ½ c. berries

Snack: Cottage cheese and veggie of choice

Lunch: Mixed greens, cucumber, tomato, and fresh dill topped with low-sodium tuna (drained) dressed with mustard; multigrain crackers

Snack: Protein Shake and veggies of choice

Snack (optional): Carrot and celery sticks with 2 t. nut butter

Dinner: Roasted Chicken and Veggies; salad dressed with olive oil and balsamic vinegar; "Baked" Apple (see recipe)

Sample Menu Eleven

Breakfast: 3 egg whites and 1 whole egg scrambled with ½ c. brown rice; mixed salad greens dressed with olive oil and lemon or orange juice

Snack: Cottage cheese and peaches

Lunch: Grilled chicken breast on a low-calorie whole wheat bun with 1 T. Avocado Spread (see recipe), lettuce, and tomato; ½ c. sliced cucumber; ½ c. grapes

Snack: 2 light string cheeses and veggies of choice

Snack (optional): Hard boiled egg and small apple

Dinner: Steak Salad (see recipe); Strawberry "Ice Cream" (see recipe)

Sample Menu Twelve

Breakfast: Protein Cookie (see recipe); 1 c. skim milk; 1 c. melon or grapes

Snack: Parfait (see recipe)

Lunch: Turkey Burger Salad (see recipe); multigrain crackers

Snack: 2 light string cheeses and veggies of choice

Snack (optional): Almonds and veggies of choice

Dinner: Grilled tilapia; Salad of mixed greens with parsley and fresh dill dressed with olive oil and lemon juice; steamed carrots; ½ c. applesauce

Sample Menu Thirteen

Breakfast: 2-3 oz. breakfast steak; 1 whole egg cooked with non-stick spray; 1 slice low-calorie whole grain bread with 1 t. grass-fed butter or heart-healthy substitute; ½ c. berries or melon

Snack: Yogurt; ½ c. sliced cucumber; multigrain crackers

Lunch: Chicken breast; ½ c. brown rice; stir-fry veggies; Asian Salad (see recipe)

Snack: Protein Shake and veggies of choice

Snack (optional): Light string cheese and small apple

Dinner: Grilled salmon; steamed broccoli; sliced tomato; mandarin oranges

Sample Menu Fourteen

Breakfast: Parfait (see recipe)

Snack: Protein Shake (see recipe); veggies of choice

Lunch: Egg Sandwich (see recipe); mixed greens salad dressed with olive oil and balsamic vinegar

Snack; Light string cheese; sliced cucumber; multigrain crackers

Snack (optional): Almonds and carrot sticks

Dinner: Italian Chicken (see recipe); ½ c. frozen blueberries (defrosted)

CHAPTER EIGHT

HEALTHY LIFESTYLE

HEALTHY LIFESTYLE

What does a healthy lifestyle look like? Does it look like a certain age, gender, or weight? Does it look like a certain style of clothes or athletic shoe? Does it look like a certain brand of "diet food" or "diet drink"? The answer is no. A healthy lifestyle looks like one healthy choice at a time. That doesn't sound so bad now, does it?

A healthy lifestyle happens when all of your healthy choices change how you think and act. By choosing to drink water instead of soda, taking the stairs instead of the elevator, eating lean proteins with lots of vegetables instead of junk food, exercising instead of sitting in front of the TV or computer, these choices add up to a healthy lifestyle.

You can't go from couch potato to athlete overnight. Start out slowly and gradually increase your activity level. You may feel like you don't know where to begin, so let me give you a few ideas. First of all, think about things that appeal to you. If the thought of jogging makes you want to reach for the cookies, then jogging wouldn't be a good choice. If, on the other hand, the thought of shooting a few hoops sounds like fun, then that is probably a better choice.

Don't be trapped into thinking that being physically active means hours on a treadmill, elliptical machine, or stationary bike. Think outside the box. There are so many things you can do. Here is a list of some activities you can try.

- rollerblading
- volleyball
- soccer
- baseball

- basketball
- hockey
- golf
- racquetball
- football
- flag football
- kickball
- batting cage
- Frisbee
- Frisbee golf
- miniature golf
- hula hoop
- swimming
- swing dance
- tap dance
- ballroom dance
- jazz dance
- hip hop dance
- belly dance
- stroll through the park
- rock climb
- white water rafting

- kayak

- ride a bike

- play catch

- skateboard

- ski

- surf

- hike

- ride a horse

- mountain bike

- box

- martial arts

- gymnastics

- ping pong

- tennis

- water aerobics

and the list goes on. There are so many things you could do; just choose one that sounds fun to you and start doing it.

Start adding more active choices to your day and you will be surprised at how easy it is. Now, don't roll your eyes at me and tell me you've heard all of this before. The reason you've heard it before and the reason I'm telling you again is because it works. Take the stairs, not the elevator. Park farther away in the parking lot instead of driving around the parking lot for ten minutes looking for the closest spot. If you need to go to the corner store to pick up one item, walk there. If you're watching television, get up and march in place or do jumping jacks during every commercial break. Take a walk on your lunch break. If you work at a desk all day, get up every hour and walk around your office (this is also a great time to drink a glass of water). Get a pedometer and challenge yourself to take more steps every day.

When you're grocery shopping, don't hunch over and lean your elbows on the shopping cart handle. Stand up straight with just your hands resting on the handle. When you push your shopping cart like that, it is not only bad for your back and posture, it makes you walk more slowly because you're steering with your elbows. Walk briskly through the store. Don't meander up and down every aisle. That's how doughnuts and chips end up in your cart. Make a menu and a list and stick to it. I mean it.

Make one healthy choice at a time and rejoice in the victory of each choice. Didn't eat one of those brownies someone brought to work? Drank all eight glasses of water today? Did your workout even when you didn't feel like it? Ate the side salad instead of the fries? Tried a new class at the gym? High five yourself, do a little victory dance, and take pride in the fact that you made a good choice.

Don't stress if you make a less than ideal choice once in awhile. Consistently making healthy choices makes a healthy lifestyle, and an occasional less-healthy choice doesn't make you "unhealthy." However, if less healthy choices happen more than your healthy choices, you need to re-evaluate your eating plan to see where you can modify it so making the healthy choice is easier. Never give up, and always look for a new path if the path you're taking isn't working for you. Each day is a new chance to make healthy choices, and each day you make healthy choices you create a healthy lifestyle.

WHERE DO YOU START?

Sometimes people will get mixed messages or confusing information on what is the best type of workout. There are some people who claim that straight up cardio is the only way to go. Others will swear by strength training. Then you have the pilates versus hot yoga crowd. There are people who claim you must work out for an hour a day, and others say to work out 30 minutes a day in three 10-minute increments spaced throughout the day. There is zone training where you try to work in a specific target heart rate zone.

There is interval training where you mix low-intensity exertion with short bouts of high-intensity exertion. There are running, biking, and tennis enthusiasts who claim that their sport of choice is the best option. Just as there are numerous opinions on healthy eating, there are just as many on exercise.

Since I am not a personal trainer I can't specifically recommend an exercise program, but I can tell you what worked for me. While I believe that *any* activity is better than no activity, I know you can't keep doing the same activity, at the same intensity, for the same duration and expect to see continued results.

You may have heard the phrase "muscle memory" thrown around in reference to workout programs. Muscle memory refers to your body's ability to learn through repetitive movement. As your body is continually exposed to repetitive movement it learns how to do the movement with maximum efficiency with as little exertion as possible. So, for those of you who continue to do the same thing over and over, your body will become more efficient and your workout will become less beneficial. For this reason you should do a variety of exercises and/or activities.

MUSCLE MEMORY TO THE EXTREME

A few short weeks after the birth of my baby I was at the gym for my workout with my trainer. I was on the elliptical for my warm-up when I suddenly woke up. No, I wasn't dreaming I was at the gym. I fell asleep while doing the elliptical. My muscles knew so well how to work the elliptical machine that when my brain fell asleep my muscles kept going. I was extremely thankful that I didn't fall off the machine, but it sure made me wish my muscle memory included getting a full night's sleep.

I do a combination of many activities. I do elliptical, stationary bike, strength training (always working different muscle groups), walking and running on both the treadmill and outside, laps in the pool, water aerobics, exercise DVDs, running up and down the stairs at home, hula hoop, and dance. I constantly challenge myself to do or learn new things. One week of workouts may look like this:

Monday: Water aerobics.

Tuesday: Personal trainer followed by walking on the treadmill or swimming laps.

Wednesday: Core exercises and some running or intervals on the treadmill.

Thursday: Strength training and treadmill or pool.

Friday: Dancing.

Saturday: Walk in the park with the kids.

Sunday: Day of rest.

You may have noticed that I had a day of rest in my workout schedule. Just as a good night's sleep is important for recovery, so is a day of rest. Your body needs time to recover, so one day of rest a week is a good idea.

If you consistently push yourself without giving your body a break, you run the risk of over-training. You may think that going full speed ahead every day will get you better and quicker results, but if you start to over-train the opposite is true. When you over-train, it destroys your metabolism and your body stops using fat for fuel. When your body stops using fat for fuel it becomes increasingly difficult to not only lose fat but to lose weight in general. So all of your hard work isn't going to give you the results you desire. Take it easy and give yourself a break once a week. Trust me; you're going to need it.

Now, how do you start incorporating more activity into your day? Do it gradually and it will be easier to do. Try adding some walking to your day; it is easy, convenient, and you don't need any special equipment to do it. Try doing any activity that appeals to you. Don't try to tell me you can't find *one* activity you like. When you find something, just start doing it in short increments of time and gradually build up your endurance. You can try doing some low-intensity cardio such as the stationary bike, treadmill, or elliptical machine. Start out slowly (remember, I started out doing only 10 minutes), do what you feel you can do, and slowly increase it. Try a class at the gym, an exercise DVD, or working with a personal trainer if you want more structure.

The main thing is to consistently do a workout or activity. By consciously trying to incorporate more activity into your day you will quickly reap the benefits of an active lifestyle: more energy, improved cardiovascular function, lower stress levels, improved sleep, improved strength, and weight loss.

If you are only doing something active once a week you're not going to achieve the benefits as quickly as you may want.

NO PAIN NO GAIN

I think we've all heard the saying "no pain, no gain," and, to a certain extent, that is true. Sore muscles mean you worked your muscles, but sharp or persistent pain should never be ignored. There is a big difference between the customary soreness from strength training or intense cardio training and the pain of an injured muscle or joint. Always listen to your body. If something doesn't feel right, pay attention. An overworked muscle is prone to injury.

If you sustain an injury it typically takes 6-8 weeks to recover. During that time you will need to modify your workout accordingly. You should seek medical care and follow the guidelines of your healthcare provider. If you are working with a trainer, you must let them know about your injury and any restrictions you have.

Now, don't be getting all nervous about getting hurt if you work out. The risks associated with obesity far outweigh the risk of a pulled muscle. If you are smart about working out and always warm-up, stretch, and cool-down you will decrease your risk. You may think that doing those things sounds boring or will take up precious time that you don't have, but, trust me, they are the most important things you can do to avoid injury.

Once you start working out you will get sore. It comes with the territory. If you're using your muscles in a whole new way, they protest a little bit. It is important to keep moving to keep the muscle aches at a minimum. If you feel like working out will be too much, you can at least do some stretching and slow walking to keep your muscles loose. Muscle soreness peaks the second day after a workout, so don't be alarmed if you feel pretty good the first day after a workout and really sore the second day.

If you are so sore after a workout that you can hardly move for a few days, you need to evaluate why. Did you forget to warm-up, stretch, and cool-down? Did you not warm-up long enough? Did you lift weights that were too heavy? Excessive soreness that disrupts your workout schedule doesn't help you at all, and, in that case, the "no pain, no gain" motto is ridiculous. If you're working with a trainer whose sole objective is to make you sore, you probably need a new trainer.

REAL LIFE TRAINING

Working with a trainer is perhaps not what most people think it is. Due to the popularity of reality television programs that show people working with trainers who are super intense—yelling, in your face, showing no mercy as their client is on the verge of collapse—there is a misconception that personal trainers are similar to drill sergeants. While there may be personal trainers like that out there, I have yet to meet one.

Every personal trainer will have their own training style, so it is important to find a trainer who will work well with you. Some people may want that kind of intense, drill sergeant type of trainer. Others may want someone with a strong sense of empathy to hold their hand every step of the way. A trainer who is adept at teaching may be better for still others. Whichever style of training encourages, motivates, and helps you reach your goals is the best style for you. For myself, I prefer a trainer with a strong teaching component, who constantly encourages me to do better, helps me stay focused, and doesn't mind my constant questions, all while holding me accountable.

Most trainers will have a set plan of what they will be working on with their client before their session, but because my trainer can never anticipate how I might be doing he has to have a couple options ready. A personal training session with my trainer usually starts with my trainer asking me how I'm feeling. Technically, he usually asks, "How's your head?" If I'm having trouble with my dizziness it will impact what type of workout we'll do. If I'm having a migraine we typically will avoid any floor work or anything with excessive movement. If I'm recovering from a migraine we will usually do a lot of balance work. If I'm feeling fine he just kicks my butt, for serious.

So, what does a butt-kicking look like? It is being pushed as far as you can be. It is doing better, with more intensity, lifting heavier, working harder, and accomplishing more than you ever thought you could do. If I'm working out on my own, I may pick up a weight and think, "That's heavy," and set it down and get a lighter weight. If I'm working out with my trainer and he gives me a weight and I say, "That's heavy." He says, "I know, now lift it," and I do. If I ever start to falter he always tells me, "You're okay," and usually that is all I need to get me through.

Sometimes, he has to stay right with me verbally. "Come on, now. You can do it." Every once in awhile he has to use his "trainer" voice on me. Doing some intense power training, he had me chest pressing a baby elephant and I made the mistake of saying, "I can't." He had his "trainer" voice on in an instant. "Don't ever say you can't! Say you're having trouble lifting this weight." Sufficiently chastised, I replied, "Sorry, I don't know what I was thinking. Probably due to the lack of oxygen going to my brain because I was trying to lift such a heavy weight."

My training session is not going to look like anyone else's training session, because it is *my* training session. That is why it is called personal training; my session is for *me*, not for anyone else. I'm not competing against anyone at the gym but myself, so I can't compare myself to anyone else at the gym. I can't look at the weight I'm lifting and compare it to the weight some guy half my age and twice my height is lifting. I can't compare the speed at which I'm running on the treadmill to the speed of someone old enough to be my mother. All I can do is do the best for me.

MY DAY

One day I was headed to the gym, late as usual. I pulled into the parking lot and realized someone was parked in *my* spot. Bummer. Dropped my kids off in the child center and headed to the locker room, only to discover that someone was using *my* locker. Darn it. Got dressed and started for the treadmill for some extreme intervals and the lady walking ten feet ahead of me took *my* treadmill. Really? Finished the intervals and went to the pool to cool down with some laps. Hung my towel up and knocked out twenty laps, got out of the pool and saw that someone had taken *my* towel. Guess it wasn't *my* day.

WHAT'S SO BAD ABOUT THE GYM?

I see all kinds of weight loss infomercials that say, "And you don't have to go to the gym!" My question is: what's so bad about the gym? I'm not sure why, or how, going to the gym came to be viewed so negatively. Perhaps it is the fear of the unknown, perhaps it is the misconception that the gym is full of big, burly guys whose bicep circumference is bigger than their IQ, or perhaps it is just an excuse that people will use to avoid getting in shape. Whatever the reason, I am here to tell you that the gym is not a scary place; it is an amazing tool that you can use to help you reach your goals.

No, I'm not a trainer, and I don't work at a gym, but sometimes I feel like I live there. I am one of a rare breed of people who enjoys working out. It wasn't always that way. For the longest time, I was extremely intimidated by the gym. Embarrassment, self-consciousness, and insecurity kept me far away.

Once I got there, I was so glad I had summoned the courage to go. The gym became a great place for me to learn and a great place for me to find support and friendship. To me, the sights, sounds, and smells of a gym are as comforting as my own home. The gym is where I enjoy "me time," not having to worry about the dishes or laundry that needs to be done, what I'm making for dinner, or whatever demands there are on my schedule. It is where I go to relax and unwind. Pretty weird, huh?

I would like to encourage you to let go of any excuses, insecurities, or embarrassment that are keeping you from seeking out a gym. Find the courage that I didn't have and go for it! There are so many resources available to you there, resources that will help you achieve success on your weight loss journey and reach your health and fitness goals.

GYM RAT

I don't understand why being interested in health and fitness is viewed so negatively. If you are watching your nutrition and trying to eat healthy, you're a "health nut." If you enjoy being physically fit and active, you're a "fitness freak." If you work out at a gym, you're a "gym rat." I say, keep your negativity to yourself because not only do I bear the name "gym rat," I wear it with honor.

Now, you may be asking yourself how you know if you're a gym rat. I've put together an easy checklist so you can determine if you're a real gym rat or not. Just make sure you're not a gym jerk.

<u>YOU'RE A GYM RAT IF:</u>

- Your gym bag weighs at least 10 pounds.

- You carry the lingering scent of chlorine from the pool.

- You use your gym membership card more than your debit card.

- Half of your friends on Facebook are people from the gym.

- You get upset if someone uses "your" locker, or parks in "your" spot.

- At least 50% of your wardrobe is workout clothes.

- You have a gym membership at more than one gym.

- You won't pay $15.00 for a pair of jeans, but you will pay $20.00 for workout shorts.

- Not only the staff, but other gym members know your workout routine.

- You get in the car to run an errand and automatically drive to the gym.

- Your trainer knows your menstrual cycle better than your husband.

- 90% of the staff at the gym recognizes you by sight, and 50% know you by name.

- You can easily spend 2 hours at the gym.

- You know the difference between "reps" and "sets."

- Water from the pool randomly pours out of your ear when you're sleeping.

- You have actually had sweat drip off your body.

- You have your gym bag packed and are halfway to the gym before you finish reading a text asking if you want to go work out.

- You get a text asking if you want to go to the gym, and you're already there.

- You carry protein and/or food in your gym bag.

- You kind of like the smell that comes out of the men's locker room.

<u>YOU'RE NOT A *REAL* GYM RAT IF:</u>

- You're reading a book during your workout.

- You're wearing jeans and a flannel button down shirt.

- You're not sweating.

- You have only used one piece of equipment since you joined the gym.

- You actually listen to the music they play at the gym.

- Your gym bag has wheels.

- Your gym shoes still have the price tag on.

- You think using the sauna counts as a workout.

- You still look cute after your workout.

- You're a woman and you don't wear a sports bra.

- You're a man and you need a sports bra.

- You have never grunted, groaned, panted, grimaced, or cursed during a workout.

<u>YOU'RE A GYM JERK IF:</u>

- You don't put equipment back when you're done.

- You come to the gym sick and spread your germs on the equipment.

- You just drop the weights after your set, instead of putting them down.

- You yell like a crazy person while lifting.

- You don't wipe your sweat off the equipment.

- You talk on the phone while at the gym.

- You stay on one piece of equipment forever and don't let anyone else have a turn.

- You get in the pool or hot tub without rinsing off first.

- You join someone in the pool lap lane without asking first.

- Your gym offers towel service and you use more than one towel.

- You use the bathroom stall to change your clothes.

- You check out members of the opposite sex.

- You check out yourself in the mirror.

CHAPTER NINE

COMMON CONCERNS

THE SKINNY ON GETTING SKINNY

I know that you have questions about what it's really like when you lose weight. There are a lot of questions, concerns, fears, myths, excuses, and misconceptions out there regarding weight loss. No question or concern is too small. If it is important to you then it deserves to be addressed. So let's get started.

I'm afraid that if I lose weight I will have lots of excess sagging skin. This is a very common, legitimate, and valid concern. Some people would rather be heavy than risk having excess sagging skin. I lost weight in a slow, steady, healthy, and safe manner while toning through weight training, and I was lucky enough to have enough elasticity in my skin to not have trouble with excess skin, but I know women who have had this problem. There is no way you can predict if you will have saggy skin. Whether or not you get saggy skin after losing weight is dependent on many factors, such as how heavy you are, how long you've been heavy, skin elasticity, age, and rate and method of weight loss. If you are extremely heavy, have been heavy for a very long time, have lost and regained weight repeatedly, lose weight rapidly (more than 2 pounds a week), or lose weight in an unhealthy manner, your chances of encountering this issue will increase. Try to lose weight in a safe and healthy manner through proper diet and exercise at a steady rate of no more than 2 pounds a week, and tone up through weight training or resistance training to decrease your chances of saggy skin.

Will my breasts shrink when I lose weight? Now, for some people the thought of smaller breasts has them dreaming of all of the cute little bras that they have always been too large-busted for. For others, the thought of losing what little they have been endowed with is an unwelcome possibility. Growing up I had always been large busted, with a lot of boys at school razzing me about the size of my breasts. As I got heavier with and breastfed each baby, my breasts responded accordingly by getting larger and larger, as high as 40F (F for Freaking Huge!). I had always looked longingly at the cute little bras and wished they made them in my size. As I lost weight, a lot of those cute little bras were suddenly my size and, I must admit, I had quite a bit of fun buying matching little bra and panty sets. While it was fun to finally be able to buy the cute bras, it was a little disconcerting to watch my womanly assets disappear. Breasts are made of fat and when you lose weight, you lose fat, *wherever* it is on your body. So, yes, your breasts will shrink, but you can tone your chest muscles and invest in a good bra to show off what you still have.

I just found the cutest jeans two sizes smaller than what I wear. Should I buy them as "Goal Jeans"? This is a dangerous question. It is vital to always have a goal to be striving for, but sometimes "goal jeans" can be the worst thing in the world. After having my surprise baby, I wanted to get my body back as quickly as possible. I wanted to wear my clothes, I didn't want to buy "fat clothes," and, no matter what the salespeople at the maternity store say about how you can wear your maternity clothes after you have the baby, I didn't want to wear maternity clothes under any circumstances. I gave in and bought a pair of jeans, just so I had something to wear, and found another pair on clearance for $3.00 in the next size smaller that I decided to get as "goal jeans." I would try on the goal jeans every once in awhile to see if they fit me yet. I knew the baby weight was coming off and I felt like I was looking better, but I could not fit into those jeans. I got increasingly frustrated as all of my efforts to fit into those goal jeans did not get me any closer to zipping them up. One day, I was walking through the thrift store and saw a cute pair of jeans that looked like they would fit, so without looking at the size or trying them on I bought them. When I got home I tried them on and, much to my delight, they not only fit but they were cute, too. Then I looked at what size they were: childrens 16. What?! How could that be? I had been trying for weeks to zip up my junior's size 9 "goal jeans" with no luck, but the childrens 16 fit perfectly. I held the two jeans up together and the "goal jeans" were smaller than the childrens jeans. They were sized incorrectly; no wonder they were on clearance. For weeks I had been feeling frustrated and upset because I couldn't fit into my "goal jeans," fearing that I would never get my body back. I let my inability to fit into those stupid jeans color the way I felt, and the way I felt I looked. Just because the tag on those jeans said a particular number, that tag did not make those jeans that size. Don't let a size on a tag cloud your thinking. Buy clothes that fit well regardless of what the number on the tag says. If you feel like you absolutely *must* have the cute pair of jeans as a goal, be aware that they may never fit the way you want and buy with caution. Whatever you do, don't be tempted to squeeze into a size that really doesn't fit you just to say you're a certain size. Wearing clothes that are too tight or too small will not make you look thinner; they will make you look fatter. You will have rolls of fat that need to find a place to go because they won't fit into those too small jeans, and where those rolls of fat end up is usually in a very unflattering place. I'll let you in on a little secret. No one knows what the tag inside your jeans says, so instead of stressing over what random number is on that silly little tag, look in the mirror and see how nice you look in a pair of jeans that fit you properly.

I have heard that when you lose weight you will get an increase in your libido. Is that true? Surprise sixth baby. Enough said.

Only divas work with a trainer. False. Lots of people work with trainers: young people, old people, males, females, athletes, people overcoming injury or surgery, healthy people, people trying to get healthy, people trying to lose 20 pounds, people trying to lose 100 pounds. Anyone can work with a trainer, and having a trainer does not mean you're a diva. Anyone that is interested in becoming more physically fit can benefit from working with a trainer. Trainers can not only teach you exercises, they can teach you the proper form for performing exercises, put an exercise routine together for you to meet your specific needs, give advice and encouragement, and help guide you on your path to health and fitness.

I don't want to lift weights because I don't want to get too muscular. This is a common concern for a lot of women, so let me clarify: weight training is not the same as bodybuilding. Bodybuilding is where you get very muscular and drop your body fat extremely low to see the definition of muscles, and is usually done for competition. Weight training is using (lifting) weights to tone muscle, increase strength, increase bone density, improve flexibility, and increase anaerobic endurance. The main difference between the two is the amount of weight and the number of reps utilized. Bodybuilders will typically lift very heavy weights with low reps to increase muscle mass. Weight training is lifting a lighter weight at higher reps to tone and strengthen. For example, if I am trying to tone my arms (weight training) I might do fifteen bicep curls with five pounds; if I am trying to increase the size of my bicep (bodybuilding) I might do eight bicep curls with twenty pounds. Trust me, the people that do bodybuilding have to work extremely hard to look the way they do. You will not "accidentally" get too muscular.

I keep hearing the words "reps" and "sets." What do they mean and what's the difference? Good question. People that are familiar with working out throw these words around carelessly, not realizing that a lot of people don't know what they mean. The word "reps" is short for "repetitions." A repetition is how many times you do something. A "set" is a group of repetitions. Let's say you're doing crunches. You may do three sets of fifteen reps, which is doing fifteen crunches (reps) and then taking a short rest period at the end to finish the set, then fifteen crunches and a short rest for the second set, and finally fifteen crunches with a rest period at the end of the last (third) set for a total of forty-five crunches.

I keep doing crunches but I can't get rid of my belly fat. What am I doing wrong? What you're doing wrong is thinking wrong. You have fallen victim to the myth that doing crunches makes belly fat disappear and that, unfortunately, is not how it works. You could do a hundred crunches every day and have fabulous muscle tone, but not be able to see it because of belly fat. Losing belly fat, for women, is not necessarily the easiest thing to do. There are nine primary fat deposit areas on women, and one of those areas is around the navel, which is why even thin women who have never had children can still have an issue with belly fat. In order to lose belly fat you need to drop your overall body fat percentage, and this is where it gets tricky. If you drop your body fat percentage too low you run the risk of developing hormonal problems like amenorrhea, which is a temporary absence of ovulation with resulting absence of menstrual cycle and loss of fertility. When you see women with extremely low body fat percentages, be aware that their appearance comes with a price. If your body fat percentage is at a level that can be safely reduced, a healthy diet is going to be your most effective weapon in the battle of belly bulge. Try to keep your fat intake at no more than 30% of your overall calories, make sure your caloric intake is sufficient (too few calories leads to the body storing fat) but not excessive, and drink plenty of water to flush away all the fat. Continue to do crunches, so when your belly fat disappears you will look toned and fabulous.

I'm going to the gym and trying to get healthy, but my friend said I'm being selfish. What should I do? Women are supposed to be self-sacrificing, putting everyone's needs before their own, regardless of the politically correct statement, "You need to take care of yourself first, so you can take care of everything else." A lot of women struggle with guilt if they can't do everything they think they're supposed to be doing, which is why most women say they are too busy to go to the gym. If you have decided to get healthy and are making going to the gym one of your priorities, you are most definitely not being selfish. You are the victim of a saboteur. Your friend is operating out of jealousy and insecurity, trying to undermine your healthy efforts. Don't let this person sway your determination to do what needs to be done to reach your health goals. Turn a deaf ear to their derogatory whisperings and continue on your journey of health and fitness.

Help! I've hit a plateau in my weight loss; what do I do now? First of all, congratulate yourself for taking the steps necessary to lose enough weight to hit a plateau. Now, calm down and let me explain something to you. Hitting a plateau is not necessarily a bad thing. A plateau in weight loss is a sign that your metabolism is shifting gears. You have modified your eating and activity levels enough for your metabolism to decide it needs to change. This is not the time to give up or do some weird, crazy diet trick. Give yourself a few weeks to let your metabolism figure out what it's doing while you continue doing what you've been doing. After a few weeks you can change either your eating or your activity levels, or both. If you've been eating 2000 calories a day you may want to try eating 1800 calories instead. If you've been walking on the treadmill for 30 minutes a day three times a week you might want to replace one treadmill day with strength training. It is possible to plateau more than once during your weight loss journey as your metabolism continues to adjust. If it happens again, just relax and pat yourself on the back for giving your metabolism a wake-up call.

Thin people are healthy. I know that at first glance this myth appears to be true, but being thin does not equal being healthy. Some thin people struggle with various illnesses that make them thin, some thin people struggle with eating disorders, some thin people suffer from heart disease, high blood pressure, and high cholesterol. There are some thin people who only eat junk food and never exercise who have as much trouble tackling a flight of stairs as an overweight person. Just because someone appears thin to you does not mean that their underlying health is good, and so it's also true that just because someone isn't model thin doesn't mean they are unhealthy. Health is measured in a lot of ways: healthy cholesterol levels, normal blood pressure, cardiovascular health, absence of illness or disease processes, and healthy weight. As I was losing weight, I ate very healthy and exercised regularly, and even though I still looked heavier, I was in better shape than a lot of people who might have looked thinner than me. So this notion of "thin is healthy" isn't entirely true.

My medication makes it hard for me to lose weight. This is a tough one. When I suffered from my illness I was prescribed a lot of medications that had "weight gain" as a side effect. Ironically a lot of them also had dizziness as a side effect too (go figure), so I know how difficult this one is to deal with. Medications, including birth control pills, can make it difficult to lose weight, but that doesn't mean weight loss is impossible. You may have to be more patient on your weight loss journey and accept the fact that it may take you a little longer to get where you want to be. Trust me, the view in your mirror will be just as amazing, no matter how long it takes you to get there.

You can't eat when you're losing weight. This one always makes me laugh, because I'm *always* eating. I think I eat more frequently than my newborn baby. I eat every 2-3 hours; if I go longer than 3 hours I feel like I'm going to pass out. I always have food with me, just in case an errand takes too long and I can't get home to eat. I keep food in my purse, in my gym bag, and I often have an insulated lunch sack with a snack in it with me. The key to losing weight is eating small frequent meals, so you're never overly hungry or overly full. Eating every couple of hours is a great way to speed up your metabolism, and the better your metabolism, the easier it is to lose weight. So don't be afraid to eat; just make sure you're making the healthiest choice you can.

I'm too old to get healthy. Don't believe this. It is *never* too late to start taking care of your health.

If I eliminate all fat from my diet I will lose weight. This is a common, but dangerous misconception. Eliminating food groups is a dangerous practice, even if the food group is fat. The human body needs fat in order to function properly. The body needs healthy fats like those found in nuts, avocados, fish oils, olive and coconut oils as part of a healthy diet. What the body does not need is an excessive amount of deep-fried fatty foods, so put down the deep-fried candy bar.

I can't afford a gym membership. Cost can be a big deterrent for many people, so let me encourage you to look at all of your options. There are many different types of gyms that offer a wide variety of fitness options at lots of different prices. Do a little research and see what gym meets your needs the best, and then see what options they have for membership. Then honestly look at your budget. If you give up your $5.00 a day coffee, can you afford the gym?

I don't have time to go to the gym. Time is another factor that people really have issues with. It seems like there are never enough hours in a day. People always ask me how I find time to go to the gym and my answer to that is that I *make* time to go to the gym because it is a priority for me. I encourage you to honestly look at how you spend your time. If your "busy" evening consists of you sitting in front of the TV watching your favorite shows or checking out your Facebook, perhaps you're not as "busy" as you think.

A lot of people think you have to go to the gym at the crack of dawn and work out first thing in the morning. Not true. As a busy mom, the best time for me to go to the gym was in the evening after most of my kids were settled down for the night. When one of my kids took a conditioning class at the gym, I switched my workouts to the same time since I was already at the gym. When I was pregnant, I had to change my workouts and that meant taking some water aerobics classes in the morning. Going to the gym and staying fit and healthy are major priorities for me, so I do what I need to do to fit it into my schedule.

You need to find a time that works for you. You might work near a gym so you can go workout at lunch or right after work. Maybe working out in the middle of the afternoon so you can avoid the crowds is easier for you. Or maybe you don't mind working out first thing in the morning and you enjoy starting your day off with a good workout to motivate and inspire you to make healthy choices the rest of the day. Do what works for you, and be aware of your changing needs. If your work schedule changes, or it's summer and the kids aren't in school anymore, you may need to adjust when you work out. Be flexible, and be honest about where your time is spent. If your health is a priority for you, you will be surprised to find that you have plenty of time to go to the gym.

The gym is only for people that are fit. If you're not going to the gym because you think everyone there is fit, let me assure you that that is simply not true. Yes, there are fit people at the gym, but there are people in every stage of health and fitness there as well. There are people just starting out on their journey, there are people who are well on their way towards meeting their goals, people who are coming back after a detour, and people who have reached their initial goals and are working towards new goals. The gym is for *everyone,* no matter where they are in their journey.

I don't know how to work the equipment at the gym. If you are intimidated by the equipment at the gym, don't panic. Gyms typically offer some type of free "orientation" where you can learn about the equipment and ask questions regarding any personal concerns you may have. Gym equipment always has instructional information on the equipment itself in case you forget. If all else fails, just ask someone if you don't know or don't remember how something works. Gyms are filled with personal trainers that are there to help answer any questions you may have. Don't be embarrassed to ask for help; that is how you learn. You never know, stopping to ask for help may introduce you to a personal trainer who just might be a perfect fit for you.

I don't understand gym etiquette. If you've never been to a gym before you may be concerned about how a gym really works. Gym etiquette is definitely something you need to know. A big concern people, especially women, have is the fact that gyms are notorious for being "pick-up" joints. While this can be true, there are some gyms where that type of thing is more prevalent. Generally speaking, a family-friendly gym will have less of that than an "adults only" gym. Either way, a good rule of thumb is to avoid eye contact with members of the opposite sex.

I highly recommend dressing appropriately for the gym. Ladies should always wear a sports bra, no exceptions! A built-in bra does not count as a sports bra. If you are larger busted or just want extra support, wear two sports bras. If you're going to be doing anything on the floor, wear tight fitting bottoms either alone or under loose fitting shorts, or wear long pants. Try to wear black; light colors like white or pastels tend to get see-through when you're sweating. Gray shows *exactly* where you are sweating so try not to wear gray bottoms. Wear workout clothes that wick away moisture (sweat) so you can work out more comfortably. Do not wear street clothes or street shoes. Get a good pair of shoes and some workout clothes that fit you well (not too tight and not too loose).

It is okay to ask someone if they're done with a piece of equipment that you want to use. Just wait until they're done with their set. Generally, if someone is circuit training they may put a towel or water bottle by a piece of equipment to "save" it for them. In that case, just ask if you can rotate in and use the equipment when they're resting between sets. If you want to share a lap lane in the pool, always ask if you can share before you just join someone in their lane.

LET THE JOURNEY BEGIN

The journey of health and fitness is just around the corner and I encourage you to take the first step. Yes, it's scary. Yes, it's hard. Yes, it's worth it. It is *so* worth it. Decide to get healthy, choose your method for getting healthy, deal with your emotional issues (or at least admit they're there), change your diet gradually, start moving, get your support system in place and you *will* succeed.

I have addressed your concerns, debunked the myths, pulled the plug on your excuses and taken the mystery out of how a gym works. Given you a strategy to help you change how you eat and provided options for increasing your activity levels. Encouraged you to set realistic, attainable goals and surround yourself with support. The rest is up to you. I know you can do it, and I look forward to seeing you at the gym.

CHAPTER TEN

RECIPES

PROTEIN SHAKES

Original Power-cino

This is the first protein shake I ever made. This recipe became the building block for my culinary imagination. Little did I know when I made this protein shake how many recipe ideas would come from it. For those coffee aficionados who cringe at the thought of using instant coffee, you can use some of your favorite brewed coffee in place of the milk or water and instant coffee. Just make sure the coffee has cooled down to room temperature.

8 oz. water or skim milk

2 T. instant coffee

1/2 t. unsweetened cocoa powder

1 t. vanilla extract

1 scoop vanilla protein powder

½ c. ice

Place all ingredients except ice in blender and blend until all protein powder is incorporated. Add ice and blend until smooth.

Mint Mocha Protein Shake

When I first started making power-cinos, they tasted like the average frozen coffee drink you can get at any coffee house. That made me think of my favorite coffee house drink flavor, chocolate mint, and I wondered if I could make that into a protein shake. The answer was yes, and so started the first of many protein shake recipes that began with "I wonder if...."

8 oz. water or skim milk

2 T. instant coffee

½ t. unsweetened cocoa powder

½ t. mint extract

1 t. vanilla

1 scoop vanilla protein powder

½ c. ice

Place first six ingredients in blender and blend until protein powder is well incorporated. Add ice and blend until smooth.

Chocolate, Strawberry, Banana Protein Shake

I created this recipe for my kids so they wouldn't get a caffeine rush trying to drink my power-cino. It is a favorite with both my kids and my husband. It tastes like a banana split in a protein shake.

8 oz. skim milk

1/2 t. unsweetened cocoa powder

1 t. vanilla extract

1 scoop vanilla protein powder

1/2 banana

1/2 c. frozen strawberries

Place first four ingredients in blender and blend until all protein powder is incorporated. Add fruit and blend until smooth.

Chocolate Strawberry Protein Shake

Sweet indulgence. I like to make this one around Valentine's Day since that is when everyone seems to think of chocolate-covered strawberries.

8 oz. skim milk

1/2 t. unsweetened cocoa powder

1 t. vanilla extract

1 scoop vanilla protein powder

1 c. frozen strawberries

Place first four ingredients in blender and blend until all protein powder is incorporated. Add fruit and blend until smooth.

Straight-Up Strawberry Protein Shake

Straight forward and simply delicious. A good choice for the purist who doesn't like to fuss over their food.

8 oz. skim milk

2 t. vanilla extract

1 scoop vanilla protein powder

1 c. frozen strawberries

Place first three ingredients in blender and blend until protein powder is incorporated. Add fruit and blend until smooth.

Strawberry Banana Protein Shake

Nothing is better than strawberries and bananas, except maybe strawberries and bananas blended up with some protein.

8 oz. skim milk

1 t. vanilla extract

1 scoop vanilla protein powder

1/2 banana

1/2 c. frozen strawberries

Place first three ingredients in blender and blend until protein powder is incorporated. Add fruit and blend until smooth.

Nut Butter Banana Protein Shake

This recipe creates a very rich shake, so it's perfect when you're craving something that feels like you shouldn't be eating it. For those of you that really want something decadent, try adding in ½ t. unsweetened cocoa powder.

8 oz. skim milk

1 T. nut butter

1 t. vanilla extract

1 scoop vanilla protein powder

1/2 banana

1/2 c. ice

Place first four ingredients in blender and blend until all protein powder is incorporated. Add fruit and ice and blend until smooth.

Chocolate Banana Protein Shake

Think of a banana pop all blended up so you can drink it with a straw. Yummy!

8 oz. skim milk

1/2 t. unsweetened cocoa powder

1 t. vanilla extract

1 scoop vanilla protein powder

1/2 banana

1/2 c. ice

Place first four ingredients in blender and blend until all protein powder is incorporated. Add fruit and ice and blend until smooth.

Berry Blend Protein Shake

I was inspired to make this protein shake after seeing a bag of frozen mixed berries at the store. It has amazing flavor with a heaping helping of antioxidants.

8 oz. skim milk

1 t. vanilla extract

1 scoop vanilla protein powder

1 c. frozen mixed berries

Place first three ingredients in blender and blend until protein powder is incorporated. Add fruit and blend until smooth.

Raspberry Peach Protein Shake

This is a great flavor combination that I absolutely love. If it's a little tart for your taste try adding in a little more vanilla.

8 oz. skim milk

1 t. vanilla extract

1 scoop vanilla protein powder

1/2 c. frozen raspberries

1/2 c. frozen peaches

Place first three ingredients in blender and blend until protein powder is incorporated. Add fruit and blend until smooth.

Creamsicle Protein Shake

This classic flavor reminds me of summers when I was a kid, and it always makes me smile when I drink it. I hope you enjoy it as much as I do.

8 oz. orange juice

2 t. vanilla extract

1 scoop vanilla protein powder

1/2 c. ice

Place first three ingredients in blender and blend until protein powder is incorporated. Add ice and blend until smooth.

Tropical Blend Protein Shake

This is a little taste of summer. It is perfect to sip in the summer while catching a little bit of vitamin D by enjoying the great outdoors, or on a winter day when you're dreaming of summer.

8 oz. skim milk or orange juice

1 t. vanilla extract

½ t. coconut extract

1 scoop vanilla protein powder

1 c. frozen tropical fruit blend

Place first four ingredients in blender and blend until protein powder is incorporated. Add fruit and blend until smooth.

Pineapple Whip Protein Shake

I created this recipe after trying a delicious little dessert treat while on vacation in sunny California. If you can't find frozen pineapple you can substitute with canned pineapple and a couple ice cubes to get the right consistency. If you use canned pineapple make sure the pineapple is canned in its own juice and doesn't have any sugar or artificial sweeteners added.

8 oz. skim milk

1 t. vanilla extract

1 scoop vanilla protein powder

1 c. frozen pineapple chunks

Place first three ingredients in blender and blend until protein powder is incorporated. Add fruit and blend until smooth.

Strawberry Lemonade Protein Shake

Perfect summer treat for when you want something light and refreshing to help beat the heat.

8 oz. water

1 T. lemon juice

½ t. vanilla extract

1 scoop vanilla protein powder

1 c. frozen strawberries

Place first four ingredients in blender and blend until protein powder is incorporated. Add fruit and blend until smooth.

Cherry Limeade Protein Shake

This is the unbeatable flavor of the classic cherry limeade with the extra nutritional boost of protein. This shake is a perfect example of how you can take something you enjoy and healthy it up to fit into your eating plan so you never feel like you're missing out.

8 oz. water

2 T. lime juice

½ t. vanilla

1 scoop vanilla protein powder

1 c. frozen cherries

Place first four ingredients in blender and blend until protein powder is incorporated. Add cherries and blend until smooth.

Cinnamon Vanilla Protein Shake

Two of my favorite flavors in one place. Cinnamon is a great spice that can help boost your metabolism, so I add it to a lot of my recipes.

4 oz. skim milk

4 oz. low-fat or fat-free vanilla yogurt

1 t. vanilla extract

1 t. cinnamon

1 scoop vanilla protein powder

1/2 c. ice

Place first five ingredients in blender and blend until protein powder is incorporated. Add ice and blend until smooth.

Chocolate Covered Cherry Protein Shake

Pure indulgent decadence. It tastes like you shouldn't be drinking it, because if it tastes that good it must be bad for you. This shake will turn even the most ardent holdout that thinks that if it's healthy it won't taste good into a believer. I highly recommend using almond milk in this recipe because it gives it such an amazing, rich flavor.

8 oz. skim or almond milk

1/2 T. unsweetened cocoa powder

1 t. vanilla extract

1 t. almond extract

1 scoop vanilla protein powder

1 c. frozen cherries

Place first five ingredients in blender and blend until protein powder is incorporated. Add fruit and blend until smooth.

Cherry Almond Protein Shake

Contrary to what you may be thinking, this recipe was not inspired by the scent of my lotion. Almond extract is typically added to cherry pie, which happens to be my mom's favorite. So, this one is for you, Mom.

8 oz. skim milk or almond milk

1 t. vanilla extract

½ -1 t. almond extract (to taste)

1 scoop vanilla protein powder

1 c. frozen cherries

Place first four ingredients in blender and blend until protein powder is incorporated. Add fruit and blend until smooth.

Cinnamon Peach Protein Shake

This recipe is reminiscent of a peach cobbler. A great way to feel like you're having dessert while sticking to your healthy eating plan.

8 oz. skim milk

1 t. vanilla extract

1/2 t. cinnamon

1 scoop vanilla protein powder

1 c. frozen peaches

Place first four ingredients in blender and blend until protein powder is incorporated. Add fruit and blend until smooth.

Blueberry Cinnamon Protein Shake

I know it sounds weird, but this is one of my absolute favorites. I love to have blueberries in my oatmeal with cinnamon and vanilla for breakfast, or a bowl of blueberries with a sprinkle of cinnamon and a dash of milk as "dessert" at lunch. It was only a matter of time before these flavors found their way to my blender to create this wonderful culinary masterpiece.

8 oz. skim milk

1 t. vanilla extract

1/2 t. cinnamon

1 scoop vanilla protein powder

1 c. frozen blueberries

Place first four ingredients in blender and blend until protein powder is incorporated. Add fruit and blend until smooth.

Blueberry Banana Protein Shake

Necessity is the mother of invention and that holds true for the creation of this recipe. I had half a banana I needed to use and I was out of frozen strawberries so I decided to try the banana with blueberries instead. I was pleasantly surprised by the result.

8 oz. skim milk

1 t. vanilla extract

1 scoop vanilla protein powder

1 small banana or 1/2 large banana

1/2 c. frozen blueberries

Place first three ingredients in blender and blend until protein powder is incorporated. Add fruit and blend until smooth.

Apple Cobbler Protein Shake

The recipe for this shake was inspired by a piece of chewing gum a friend of mine gave to me one day at the gym after our workout. It was one of those dessert flavor gums that I had never tried. I felt like the little girl in the 'Charlie and the Chocolate Factory' when I tasted that gum. It tasted like I was really eating apple cobbler. As soon as I tasted that gum I knew I had to make it into a protein shake. Thanks for sharing your gum and inspiring me, Mindy.

8 oz. unsweetened applesauce

2 t. vanilla extract

1/2 t. cinnamon

1 scoop vanilla protein powder

1 c. ice

Place first four ingredients in blender and blend until protein powder is incorporated. Add ice and blend until smooth.

Pumpkin Spice Protein Shake

I created this recipe when I was craving pumpkins while I was pregnant. I had a hard time finding pumpkin when I was first pregnant since it was summer and pumpkin is a seasonal item for the fall. When I was finally able to find some I was so happy, I stocked up with enough pumpkin to last me the entire pregnancy. The resulting recipe tastes like Thanksgiving and was well worth the wait. I'm betting that pumpkin will be one of my baby's favorites.

8 oz. skim milk

1 t. vanilla extract

1 t. pumpkin pie spice blend

1 scoop vanilla protein powder

1/2 c. canned pumpkin

1/2 c. ice

Place first four ingredients in blender and blend until protein powder is incorporated. Add ice and pumpkin and blend until smooth.

BREAKFAST

Low Fat Apple Cinnamon Granola

This recipe is very simple and yields a truly healthy granola. It is great by itself, with milk as a cereal, or sprinkled on a yogurt parfait.

4 c. old-fashioned oats

1 12 oz. can of frozen apple juice concentrate thawed

½- 1 T. cinnamon (to taste)

Mix all ingredients together. Spread on a cookie sheet sprayed with nonstick spray. Bake at 325° for 45 minutes, stirring every 15 minutes. Watch closely to avoid burning.

Breakfast Rice

It might sound a little weird, but it tastes great. It's a nice change from oatmeal or cold cereal.

½ c. instant brown rice, cooked

½ c. sliced strawberries

½ banana sliced

1 t. sugar

Sprinkle of cinnamon

Place freshly cooked brown rice in a bowl. Add fruit, sugar, and cinnamon and mix well.

Egg Sandwich

This recipe is perfect for breakfast or lunch. It is quick and easy to assemble so it can easily fit into your busy schedule.

1 egg white

1 whole egg

2 slices low-calorie whole grain bread

1 T. Avocado Spread (see recipe)

Sliced tomato

Lettuce

Mix egg white and whole egg together, and cook in a pan sprayed with nonstick spray. Toast the bread and top one slice with Avocado Spread, lettuce, and tomato. Add the cooked egg and the other piece of toast. Enjoy.

Avocado Spread

With healthy omega-3's, you don't have to feel guilty for wanting that creamy mouth-feel you normally get from high-fat spreads. Use this as a great, flavorful alternative to mayonnaise.

1 avocado

½ c. fat-free Greek yogurt

Lime juice to taste

Sea salt to taste (optional)

Mash avocado and stir in lime juice. Add yogurt and salt (if using), mix well. Refrigerate to keep fresh.

Breakfast Banana Split

This is so delicious, it feels like dessert instead of breakfast. One of my favorite go-to recipes.

½ c. fat-free vanilla or strawberry Greek yogurt

¼ c. granola

½ banana, "split" into two long slices

1 strawberry, diced

Put the yogurt in a bowl and place one slice of banana on each side. Sprinkle with granola and diced strawberry. Admire how beautiful it is for a brief moment before you gobble it up.

Yogurt Parfait

This is a great portable breakfast that can easily be made the night before, so there's no excuse not to have a healthy breakfast.

¾ c. fat-free Greek yogurt

½ c. diced fruit of choice

½ oz. chopped almonds

Scoop ¼ c. yogurt into a mason jar or disposable cup, layer ¼ c. fruit on top. Add another ¼ c. yogurt and ¼ c. fruit. Top with the final ¼ c. of yogurt and sprinkle with the chopped almonds. Wrap or put lid on top of fruit and yogurt and store in the fridge until ready to eat. If making the night before don't add the almonds until ready to eat.

SANDWICHES, SALADS AND SIDES

Chicken Salad Sandwich

Finally, a healthy chicken salad sandwich that isn't loaded down with fat. A light and delicious twist to a familiar favorite.

½ c. diced cooked chicken breast

½ apple, diced

2 T. diced celery

2 T. Avocado Spread (see recipe)

Freshly ground black pepper (to taste)

Alfalfa sprouts

2 slices low-calorie whole grain bread

Mix chicken breast, apple, and celery in a bowl. Add Avocado Spread and mix until all ingredients are well coated. Season with black pepper and put on one slice of bread, top with sprouts and the other slice of bread.

Tuna Salad Sandwich

A healthy-ed up version of a classic favorite. Quick and easy to prepare.

1 can low-sodium tuna, drained

2 T. diced celery

1 T. diced onion

1 T. diced carrots

2 T. diced cucumber

1 T. mustard

2 T. fat-free Greek yogurt

2 slices low-calorie whole grain bread

Throw the tuna and all the veggies in a bowl and mix to combine. Add mustard and yogurt and mix well. Assemble sandwich and enjoy.

Turkey Burger Salad

With all of the flavor of the classic hamburger, this is one of my favorite go-to meals. Perfect for lunch or dinner.

Turkey burger

2-3 c. chopped romaine lettuce

½ tomato, diced

2 T. diced onion

Mustard

Tabasco (optional)

Grill the turkey burger on George Foreman grill until thoroughly cooked (8-11 minutes). Arrange lettuce, tomato, and onion on a plate. Cut the turkey burger into bite size pieces and put on top of veggies. Drizzle with the mustard and few drops of Tabasco (if using). Delicious!

Asian Salad

Changing just a few ingredients turns a humble salad into a culinary masterpiece. This is so good I often have a second helping, for "dessert."

2 c. mixed greens

½ c. cilantro, chopped

1 green onion, sliced

½ c. small broccoli florets

1 baby carrot, sliced

1 T. seasoned rice vinegar

A few drops of sesame oil

Freshly ground black pepper, to taste

Mix salad greens and cilantro and arrange on plate. Arrange the green onion, broccoli florets, and carrot on top so it looks pretty. Drizzle with vinegar and oil and finish with the freshly ground black pepper. Super yummy!

Chicken Pasta Salad

Full of healthy nutrient-packed veggies and dressed with a fat free mayonnaise alternative, this is a guilt free way to enjoy your pasta.

½ c. cooked whole wheat pasta

½ c. diced chicken breast

½ c. small broccoli florets

2 T. diced bell pepper

2 T. diced celery

¼ c. halved grape tomatoes

¼ c. fat-free Greek yogurt

2 T. Dijon mustard

1 clove of garlic, minced

1 T. dill, chopped or 1 t. dried dill weed

Black pepper, to taste

In a medium-sized bowl, mix pasta, chicken, and all the veggies. In a separate bowl, mix yogurt, mustard, garlic, dill, and black pepper. Add yogurt mixture to pasta and toss well to coat. You can enjoy immediately or have it waiting for you at lunch.

Steak Salad

3-4 oz. cooked lean steak, sliced

2 c. chopped romaine lettuce

½ c. halved grape tomatoes

1 t. bleu cheese crumbles

1 T. Homemade "Ranch" Dressing (see recipe)

Arrange lettuce, steak, tomatoes, and bleu cheese on plate, drizzle with dressing. Season with freshly ground black pepper, if desired.

Homemade "Ranch" Dressing

A fat-free version of everyone's favorite salad dressing. Great on salad, or as a dip for your veggies. Keep a batch in the fridge so you're always ready to make a great salad.

1c. fat-free Greek yogurt

¼ c. skim milk

1 clove garlic, minced

¼ t. sea salt

1 t. sugar

1 T. dried parsley flakes

Freshly ground black pepper

Whisk yogurt and milk together in medium-sized bowl until smooth. Using the back of a knife, smash garlic and salt together to make a garlic "paste," stir into yogurt mixture. Add sugar, parsley, and black pepper, mix until ingredients are all incorporated. Refrigerate at least one hour for best flavor.

Southwest Chicken Salad

4 oz. chicken breast

½ t. garlic powder

¼ t. cumin

½ t. chili powder

2 c. chopped romaine lettuce

¼ c. chopped cilantro

1 green onion, white and green parts, sliced

1 T. fat-free Greek yogurt

2 T. salsa or picante sauce

Dice chicken breast and season with garlic powder, cumin, and chili powder. Heat sauté pan to medium-high heat and spray with nonstick spray, add chicken and cook until chicken is done (5-8 minutes). Mix lettuce, cilantro, and green onion and put on a plate, put cooked chicken on top. In a small bowl, mix yogurt and salsa or picante until smooth, drizzle over salad. You can pre-cook the chicken and keep it in the refrigerator until ready to assemble the salad for easy transport for lunch at work or, if you prefer cold chicken over hot chicken, in your salad.

Spinach Salad

A nice change from romaine lettuce or mixed greens.

2 c. chopped fresh spinach

2 T. thin-sliced red onion

½ c. halved grape tomatoes

1 t. olive oil

1 clove garlic, minced

1 T. apple cider vinegar

Freshly ground black pepper

Arrange spinach, onion, and tomatoes on a plate. Mix olive oil, garlic, and vinegar together and drizzle over the top of the salad and season with black pepper.

Garlic Green Beans

1 c. fresh or frozen green beans (defrosted)

1 t. olive oil

1 clove garlic

Freshly ground black pepper, to taste

Sea Salt (optional) to taste

Heat medium sauté pan to medium high heat, spray with nonstick spray. Add green beans and cook until desired doneness. Add olive oil and garlic and cook one more minute. Season with salt (if using) and pepper. Eat immediately for the best flavor.

Cucumber and Tomato Salad

1 cucumber, sliced

½ tomato, sliced

1 t. olive oil

1 T. apple cider vinegar

1 t. sugar

½ t. dill, chopped, or ¼ t. dried dill weed

Freshly ground pepper

Mix together cucumber and tomato. In separate bowl, whisk together oil, vinegar, sugar, and dill until sugar is dissolved. Pour over cucumber and tomato mixture. Refrigerate at least 15 minutes for best flavor, can be made up to a day in advance.

Vinaigrette Coleslaw

A healthier version of the often heavy classic side dish. This coleslaw tastes light and fresh and has a great crunch.

2 c. coleslaw mix, or shredded cabbage

2 T. apple cider vinegar

1 t. canola oil

½ t. sugar

¼ t. celery seed

Whisk vinegar, oil, sugar, and celery seed until sugar is dissolved. Pour over cabbage and mix well. Let stand 5 minutes so the cabbage wilts a bit, and stir again. Refrigerate or use immediately.

MAIN DISHES

Apricot Chicken

4 oz. chicken breast, diced

1 clove garlic, minced

¼ c. low sodium or no salt added chicken broth

2 T. chopped dried apricots

Saute chicken and garlic in a medium high pan coated with nonstick spray 3-4 minutes or until thoroughly cooked. Add chicken broth and apricots, reduce heat to low and simmer 5-8 minutes. Delicious!

Tortilla Pizza

A healthy alternative to the greasy fast food staple. Yet another example of how you don't have to give up the things you really love when you're making healthy food choices.

Low-calorie whole wheat tortilla

2 T. pasta sauce

2 T. low fat mozzarella cheese

½ c. diced cooked chicken

¼ c. diced green bell pepper

Preheat oven to 350°. Place tortilla on ungreased cookie sheet and toast in preheated oven for 5 minutes. Spoon pasta sauce on toasted tortilla and sprinkle cheese, chicken, and bell pepper evenly over tortilla. Bake 5 minutes, or until cheese is melted. Make everyone jealous by eating this in front of them.

Lemon Garlic Chicken

This is so good! Tastes light, but fills you up nicely. Quick to prepare so it's perfect for a busy weeknight.

4 oz. chicken breast

1 clove garlic, minced

1 T. lemon juice

1 T. chopped parsley

1 green onion, white and green parts sliced

Cut the chicken into bite size pieces. Heat pan to medium-high heat, spray with nonstick spray, add chicken, and cook until chicken is no longer pink in the middle. Add garlic, lemon juice, parsley, and green onion and cook one more minute. Serve immediately.

Sweet and Spicy Chicken

Sweet and spicy ranks right up there with sweet and salty on my taste buds' list of favorites. This is a simple and delicious way to have your chicken go from boring to phenomenal.

4 oz. chicken breast

½ t. garlic powder

2 T. apricot jam

¼ c. salsa or picante

Cut chicken into bite-size pieces and season with garlic powder. Heat pan to medium-high heat, spray with nonstick spray. Add chicken and cook until no longer pink in the middle, about 5 minutes. Add apricot jam and salsa or picante and cook until heated through.

Balsamic Glazed Chicken

Feels and tastes like you spent forever in the kitchen, but a truly simple way to wow your taste buds.

4 oz. chicken breast

¼ t. garlic powder

¼ t. onion powder

¼ c. balsamic vinegar

1 t. grass-fed butter or heart-healthy substitute

Cut chicken into bite size pieces and season with onion and garlic powders. Heat pan over medium-high heat and spray with nonstick spray. Add chicken and cook until almost done, approximately 3-5 minutes. Add balsamic vinegar and cook until balsamic vinegar reduces and chicken is thoroughly cooked, about 3 minutes. Add butter or butter substitute and stir until completely melted. Delicious.

Italian Chicken

A little taste of Italy. Hearty and filling, without all of the heaviness usually associated with Italian food.

8 oz. chicken breast

¼ t. garlic powder

¼ t. salt-free Italian seasoning blend

½ c. diced bell pepper (red, yellow, or green)

½ c. diced onion

1 stalk celery, diced

½ c. diced carrots

1 can no-salt-added diced tomatoes

1 T. balsamic vinegar

½ t. fennel seeds

Crushed red pepper flakes to taste

Cut chicken into bite size pieces and season with garlic powder and Italian seasoning. Heat pan to medium-high heat and spray with nonstick spray, add chicken and cook for 3 minutes. Add in the veggies and cook until chicken is thoroughly cooked and veggies are crisp tender (5-8 minutes). Drizzle with balsamic vinegar and sprinkle with fennel seeds and crushed red pepper flakes. Makes enough for two meals or two people.

SWEETS

Applesauce Protein Cookie

Since there are severe food allergies in my family, I have trouble finding protein bars that are "safe" to eat. While prepackaged protein bars are convenient, they can be high in calories and fat, and I have heard that their taste leaves something to be desired. This recipe creates a high-protein alternative without added sugar, salt, or fat. The protein I use in this recipe creates a final product with approximately 150 calories, 12 grams protein, 3.6 grams fiber, and 3.6 grams fat. It can be frozen in a zip-top sandwich bag so you can just grab it and throw it in your purse, gym bag, or lunch sack, and it tastes pretty good, too.

1 c. unsweetened applesauce

1 c. vanilla protein powder

1 egg

1 t. vanilla

1 t. cinnamon

1 c. quick cooking oats

2 T. chia seeds

Whisk together applesauce and protein until protein is well incorporated. Add egg, vanilla, and cinnamon and mix well. Stir in oats and chia seeds. Mixture will be very wet and loose. Let stand for five minutes to tighten it up a bit. Scoop onto cookie sheet sprayed with nonstick spray and bake at 375° for 10-12 minutes. Makes six extremely large cookies.

Pumpkin Spice Protein Cookie

I have to say that pumpkin is definitely something I really enjoy, so of course I found a way to put it into another recipe.

½ c. unsweetened applesauce

½ c. unsweetened canned pumpkin

1 c. vanilla protein powder

1 egg

1 t. vanilla

1 t. pumpkin pie spice

1 c. quick cooking oats

2 T. chia seeds

Mix applesauce, pumpkin, and protein until protein is well incorporated. Add in egg, vanilla, and pumpkin pie spice and mix well. Stir in oats and chia seeds. Mixture will be very wet and loose. Let stand five minutes to tighten up. Scoop onto cookie sheet sprayed with nonstick spray and bake at 375° for 10-12 minutes. Makes six huge cookies.

Banana Nut Protein Cookies

I created this recipe when I had some extra bananas. It is a healthy version of banana bread.

1 c. mashed ripe banana

1 c. vanilla protein powder

1 egg

1 t. vanilla

½ t. cinnamon (optional)

1 c. quick cooking oats

2 T. chopped nuts

2 T. chia seeds

Mix banana and protein until protein is well incorporated. Add in egg, vanilla, and cinnamon (if using) and mix well. Stir in oats, nuts, and chia seeds. Mixture will be very wet and loose; let stand five minutes to tighten up. Scoop onto cookie sheet sprayed with nonstick spray and bake in preheated oven at 375° for 10-12 minutes. Makes six deliciously humongous cookies.

Banana Chocolate Chip Protein Cookie

This is the kind of recipe that you create when you have kids who want a cookie to still feel like a treat. The chocolate chips add quite a bit more calories and fat, so don't be tempted to add more than the recipe calls for.

1 c. mashed ripe banana

1 c. vanilla protein powder

1 egg

1 t. vanilla extract

1 c. quick cooking oats

2 T. chia seeds

3 T. mini chocolate chips

Mix banana and protein until protein is well incorporated. Add egg and vanilla and mix well. Stir in oats, chia seeds, and chocolate chips. Mixture will be very loose and wet. Let stand for five minutes to tighten up. Scoop onto cookie sheet sprayed with nonstick spray and bake at 375° for 10-12 minutes. Makes six cookies the size of a toddler's head.

Strawberry "Ice Cream"

Delicious way to enjoy your fruit. The perfect treat when you "have" to have something sweet.

1 c. Frozen strawberries

¼ c. skim or almond milk

1 T. sugar

1 t. vanilla extract

Place strawberries in blender and pulse to break them down. Add vanilla and sugar and pulse a few more times to mix thoroughly. Slowly stream in the milk until the strawberries reach the consistency of soft serve ice cream. You may not need all of the milk. Enjoy immediately or put in freezer for 15 minutes to firm up.

"Baked" Apple

An absolute winner; it tastes as delicious as you hoped it would. Guilt-free dessert at its best.

1 small apple, diced

1 t. sugar

Sprinkle of cinnamon

¼ t. grass-fed butter or heart-healthy substitute

Place apple in microwave safe bowl. Add cinnamon and sugar and mix until apples are well coated. Microwave on full power in one-minute increments, stirring every minute until apples are cooked all the way through, 2-5 minutes depending on which type of apple you use. Stir in the butter or butter substitute for that taste of richness your taste buds will thank you for. Now, go enjoy it.

ABOUT THE AUTHOR

Lisa is a busy mother of six who turned her life around by embracing a healthy lifestyle. Her transformation led her to become a passionate advocate about all things health and fitness related. She lives in the beautiful state of Colorado where she enjoys maintaining her active lifestyle by competing in 5ks, triathlons, and half-marathons. Taking full advantage of the many trails to hike, bike and run on.

The writing of this book is from one "regular" person to another, based on her own experience. Since writing the book she has gone on to receive the following certifications:

NESTA Lifestyle & Weight Management Specialist

Precision Nutrition Level 1

NASM Personal Trainer

Beachbody Cize Live!

RESOURCES

Nutritional Counseling and Personal Training

Lisa Virgil

fattogymrat@gmail.com

FaceBook: Fat To Gym Rat

www.vitalizehealthandfitness.com

FaceBook: Vitalize Health And Fitness

Chiropractic and Homeopathic Health

Dr. Michael Valier 719.260.9611

Dr. Jessica Valier 719.282.2109

www.healthunlimitedcolorado.com

Graphic Design

AJ Virgil 719.200.5545

www.ajvirgil.com

Gyms

www.lifetimefitness.com

www.24hourfitness.com

www.ymca.net

www.goldsgym.com

www.ballyfitness.com

www.snapfitness.com

www.fitness19.com

www.fitnessfirst.com

www.anytimefitness.com

www.villasport.com

www.planetfitness.com

www.lafitness.com

www.curves.com

SPECIAL THANKS

Special thanks and a huge shout-out to Jen Keating and Sara Schafer. To Jen for her endless patience with my constant interruptions to her work to ask her opinion and for her honest answers to my endless questions. To Sara for her willing and helpful attitude, her attention to detail and her extra set of eyes for when I could no longer "see" my book. Many thanks, ladies!